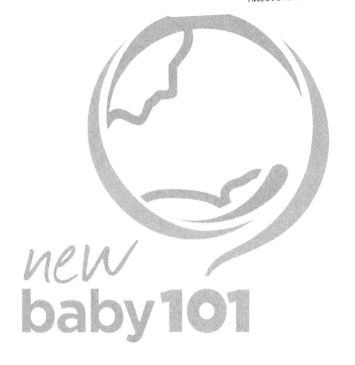

new baby 101

A Midwife's Guide For New Parents

Everything you need to know
about your New Baby

Lois Wattis

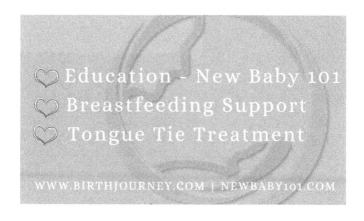

♡ Education - New Baby 101
♡ Breastfeeding Support
♡ Tongue Tie Treatment

WWW.BIRTHJOURNEY.COM | NEWBABY101.COM

Join us on Facebook

newbaby101 Facebook page

First edition published in 2014 © Lois Wattis 2022
Second edition published in 2017 © Lois Wattis 2022

This edition (3rd) published in 2022
Copyright © Lois Wattis 2022

ISBN: 978-0-6453938-1-1 (pbk)
ISBN: 978-0-6453938-0-4 (ebk)

Cover image: Evalyn © Megan Willis Photography 2022

Third edition published with the assistance of:
Publicious Book Publishing
www.publicious.com.au

Contents

New Baby 101 "How to" videos

To watch New Baby 101 "How To" videos visit: www.NewBaby101.com.au.

or scan the QR Code below:

NewBaby101 Youtube channel

Application of Nipple Shield

How to fold cloth nappies

How to change baby's nappy

How to bath baby

How to latch and breastfeed a newborn

How to swaddle your baby

How to breastfeed your baby

Introducing Lois

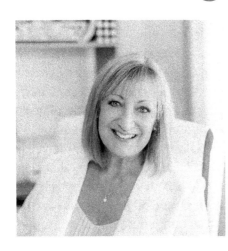

LOIS WATTIS IS A REGISTERED MIDWIFE, International Board Certified Lactation Consultant and a Fellow of the Australian College of Midwives. Working in both hospital and community settings, Lois enhanced her skills and expertise by providing woman-centered care as an Independent Practising Midwife to hundreds of mothers and babies, including more than 50 women who chose to give birth at home.

Lois' passionate approach to birth and breastfeeding nurtures women's inborn mothering instincts, supporting and enabling them to make informed choices. Lois' advanced skills as a Clinical Lactation Consultant have helped thousands of mothers in acute hospital settings and via her private Lactation Consultancy service on the Sunshine Coast, Queensland. **www.birthjourney.com**

Lois is eminently qualified to offer advice and support to new parents via her **New Baby 101 Book**. Lois is the author of numerous articles and professional guidelines which have been published in parenting magazines and midwifery journals in Australia, New Zealand and the UK. All advice provided in **New Baby 101** is based on reliable evidence and research, and Lois's common-sense approach will both inform and reassure parents as they gain new skills and confidence during the first few months of baby's life.

FOREWORD
By Pinky McKay

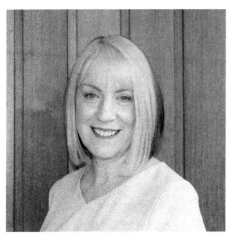

HAVING A BABY IS EXCITING and wonderful but it can also be completely overwhelming, especially when you are bombarded by advice from all directions – even from perfect strangers! It can be difficult to choose which advice to follow, especially if you already have a brand new baby. Your changing brain and body chemistry, which are nature's way of helping you adapt to the enormous job of nurturing your baby, mean that you aren't in a space where you can absorb complicated instructions. That is where **New Baby 101 Book** comes in.

Lois Wattis is not only a brilliant midwife and lactation consultant with a wealth of experience, she is also a mother and grandmother. You will be reassured by her sensible, practical advice and her calm voice. She has a very special knack of interpreting the 'medical speak' into easy language, helping you understand issues that can be frightening when they apply to your new baby. Whether you are wondering how many wees and poos your baby should be doing, how much breast-milk he is getting, how to make your baby's early tests easy and pain free or what is the latest information about jaundice, vitamin K or bonding and attachment, Lois explains your options simply, with respect, so you can make the choices that are best for your baby.

New Baby 101 Book will help you give your baby a wonderful start because it will boost your own confidence and your baby will sense this. Although it would be best to read this information before you have your baby, it will be helpful in the newborn days too. If you are feeling a little uncertain at any time, instead of looking at each other wondering 'what the hell do we do now?' a quick check will set you back on track. You will be able to relax, knowing that everything here is evidence based, written by a highly qualified health professional who cares deeply for new parents and babies. Above all, everything Lois Wattis recommends is kind and respectful to you and your baby and it will empower you to be the parents you want to be.

Love, laugh and enjoy. And please remember to be as gentle to your beloved and yourself as you are to your baby. Best wishes on this wonderful journey.

Pinky
www.pinkymckay.com

Welcome

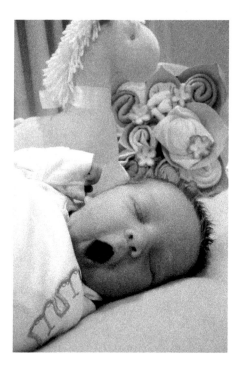

Welcome to parenting! You now have a reliable guide as you experience your "Babymoon" – the early weeks of your new life with your baby. I am sure you will find answers to your many questions in the pages which follow and you will value the practical advice I have provided.

In order to create this guide for new parents I have invested my time, my experience and my love of helping families find their own way of parenting. This is the result of my life's work as a Midwife and Mother. I trust NEW BABY 101 will help you to enjoy your journey along the steep learning curve of new parenthood.

Blessings, Lois

TOPIC 1
Before Baby is Born –
What do you *really* need?

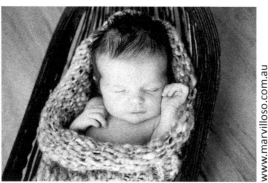

www.marvilloso.com.au

CONTRARY TO THE BABY SHOP advertisments, you actually need very little for a newborn baby. Your baby's primary needs are for closeness to his mother for warmth and comfort, breastmilk for nourishment, clean clothing, nappies/diapers and wraps and a safe place to sleep. Remember friends and family will be keen to buy your new baby gorgeous gifts to welcome him, so just buy the basic essentials when preparing for your new baby's arrival.

First and most importantly, you need to set up a **'change station'** before baby is born so it is all ready to go as this is sure to be one of the first jobs you will need to do when you get home! Watch the New Baby 101 **video "<u>How to Change Baby's Nappy/Diaper</u>"** for a practical guide. You could use a change pad on top of a chest of drawers or a table or a bench which is stable and easily accessible, or you may buy or borrow a purpose built change table with a change pad or mat. It needs to be waterproof and easy to clean as this will be the most frequently used item in your home for many months!

A clean towel or bunny rug on the surface makes it more comfortable for baby. Using water (which can be warm) and cotton balls or Chux wipes to clean baby's bottom is cheap, safe and comfortable. Use Chux or a towelling washer to dry baby's skin after cleansing. A thermos to hold some warm water is a handy addition to the change station if it is not located near a tap.

I advise parents to avoid using cleansing products such as nappy/diaper wipes on their newborn baby's delicate skin. A newborn's skin is very thin, and commercially produced baby wipes are all impregnated with chemicals of some kind, except for "**Water Wipes**" which are guaranteed to only contain water with a mild fruit extract used as a preservative.

A simple zinc and castor oil nappy cream can be used AFTER cleansing if any nappy/diaper rashes appear. Baby talcum powder is not recommended as it clogs the skin and particles can be breathed in by baby.

Two packets of 20 NEWBORN size disposable nappies/diapers will get you started. If you are interested in using cloth nappies, flannelette nappy squares can be folded smaller and are less bulky than towelling nappies on newborns. View the New Baby 101 **video "Traditional Square Nappies"** to see 5 ways to fold these to suit your baby's size and gender. **HINT:** A month's supply of flannelette nappies from a nappy wash service is a great present to have on your baby shower list.

There are also many ready-made fabric nappies with Velcro fastenings available which are comfortable for baby, but these take longer to dry after washing than traditional square nappies. Whichever nappy option you choose, it is advisable to give baby some "nappy-off time" each day to allow baby's skin to 'breathe'.

You will need a rubbish bin with a lid, and a basket for baby's soiled clothes and wraps near the change station.

NAPPY BAG

YOU WILL ALSO NEED a nappy bag stocked with nappies, water wipes, a change of clothes and spare wraps. The choices are endless, but my advice is don't get one that is enormous as you will inevitably fill it up and then it will be heavy to carry wherever you go. Take the essentials, but 'less is more'.

BABY CLOTHES

BABIES GROW VERY QUICKLY and move rapidly through the clothing sizes. A normal sized, full term baby between 3 and 4kg will fit into 0000 or 000 singlets and grow suits from birth to about 6 weeks of age. It is not good for baby to be squeezed into tight clothing – remember they are growing all the time, so it is best to always have some room to spare especially around the legs and feet.

Initially you will need 4 singlets – size 000, or smaller if you are expecting a very small baby. Growsuits or 'onesies' – get 4 in size 000, and 2 size 0000. Buy 2 little cotton hats, and 2 lightweight cardigans or jackets. If it is summer when baby is born you may prefer to get 2 growsuits without legs and feet, but you will need a couple of pairs of little baby socks. Alternately, you could buy two or three baby nighties which are very comfortable for baby boys or girls and make nappy changes really easy. This is a basic starter kit. More clothing is bound to come your way from friends and family when baby is born.

It is advisable to wash all baby's new clothes wraps and linen before use and I recommend using a gentle liquid detergent for all baby's washing. Strong washing powders and liquids can leave residual detergents in the fabrics which could irritate baby's sensitive new skin, so thorough rinsing and preferably air drying is best to protect baby's delicate skin.

Now is the time to assess your laundry equipment because it will be working overtime during baby's early months of life. You will need a reliable washing machine, and a tumble dryer is a blessing especially through the winter months. A good clothes horse will also be useful for airing and drying. Put these items on your baby shower list if you don't already have them!

BABY WRAPS

MOST NEWBORNS WILL ENJOY BEING wrapped securely (called swaddling) to settle to sleep. "Bunny Rugs" are usually made of flannelette material and are great for wrapping baby after feeds and nappy change. These can also be used as bassinet sheets. Watch the New Baby 101 video **"How to Swaddle your Baby"** for advice about safe swaddling techniques.

In warmer weather and climates bunny rugs can be replaced with Muslin wraps. These are made of a light open weave cotton so they "breathe" ensuring baby does not get too hot, and they are available in many designs. These will be handy as wraps/wipes/snugglers for many months even in cooler weather. About 6 wraps (a combination of bunny rugs and muslin wraps) should be plenty for when you bring baby home. Buy a couple of the larger sized muslin wraps as well because baby may still enjoy swaddling to settle when she grows bigger.

Ready-made swaddle suits and wraps are a popular option. Some close with Velcro and others have zips. Make sure the fabric is soft, closures are comfortable and easy to undo and the suit is not too small for your baby. It is very important that swaddles of all types are loose around baby's hips and allow baby to lift their legs and to stretch. Tight swaddling can restrict leg and hip movement and contribute to hip problems (dysplasia), so avoid sleepsuits that don't get wider from the chest downwards.

SIDS/RedNose have advised against using swaddle suits designed to position baby's arms raised upwards as they are regarded as risky if baby turns or rolls over, and concerns that restriction of arm movement could impede gross motor development and affect midline orientation. (Source: SIDS Education on-line forum 2021)

BABY BLANKETS

THE WEIGHT AND NUMBER OF baby blankets you will need depends on the season and climate. Two cotton waffle weave blankets in bassinet size will be needed whether it is summer or winter, plus one brushed cotton or wool blend warm blanket will be needed in winter. Avoid acrylic and fluffy/furry fabrics which can cause overheating and may present a SIDs risk.

SLEEP ARRANGEMENTS

BABY NEEDS A SAFE PLACE to sleep and it is strongly recommended by SIDS experts that baby sleeps in the **same room** as his parents for at least the first 6 months of life. A bassinet with a clean (preferably new) mattress, on a sturdy stand with wheels so you can move baby around the house with you is a basic item which you will need. I recommend you buy two bassinet size mattress protectors – one for your bassinet and one for your pram.

Baby could also sleep in a cot made up according to safe sleep recommendations (no bumper pads, pillows or quilts) with baby placed at the bottom of the cot and made up according to SIDS guidelines. The only disadvantage of sleeping a newborn in a cot is that it is not easily moved if desired. A baby monitor in a room is not as safe as having baby where you can easily and immediately see and hear him.

Most health authorities discourage co-sleeping (baby sleeping in the same bed as mother or parents) due to the increased risk of sleep accidents caused by baby being smothered or becoming overheated. Babies should never be slept in the same bed as a parent who smokes as the dangerous fumes exhaled by a smoker are passively breathed in by the baby. Likewise a baby in bed with anyone who is under the influence of alcohol or drugs is at great risk of harm.

However, most parents *are* likely to take their baby into bed with them at some times for feeding or cuddles to settle, and maybe to sleep, and it is unrealistic for authorities to expect or demand that this never occurs. A safe option is one of the little baby beds designed for co-sleeping, such as *The First Years* **Safe and Secure cosleeper**. These are designed to give baby a safe sleep space in the parents' bed, away from their pillows and covers.

These co-sleepers are designed so baby can be swaddled and tucked into his own little bed similar to a bassinet, but still be right beside his mother within easy reach for feeding and settling. Upright sides on the co-sleeper keep parents' bedding separate from baby, and a flap at the top tucks firmly under the parents' mattress to keep it securely in place. The co-sleeper can also be used later inside a cot to aid baby's transition from a bassinet, and it folds up to be taken with you if going out with baby. If you are non-smokers and you decide you would like to have your baby sleeping with you, even occasionally, this will be an inexpensive and worthwhile purchase. More information about safe bed-sharing is in **Topic 8 – Bedtime**.

Another option is one of the bassinets which can be attached to the side of your bed, and also convert to a freestanding bassinet. There are many choices available, and because baby outgrows a bassinet fairly quickly there are often pre-loved bargains available too.

CAR SEAT OR BABY CAPSULE

THESE ARE ABSOLUTELY ESSENTIAL ITEMS on the list if you have a car, as most people do! Baby capsules are great for small babies up to about 3 months of age, and can be hired if you prefer not to buy one. Some prams come with a capsule as a first option. A baby capsule is fine for baby for the first few months and not needing to wake baby to transfer him from the car to where ever you are going is a big advantage.

If you are using a car seat from birth you will need to handle baby to strap her in and probably waken her each time you transfer her in and out of the car. The car seat or capsule fittings should be positioned on the passenger-side of the car so the parent is not at risk of being struck by a passing car when outside of the car. It is surprising how many parents put the baby's seat on the driver's side as it seems more convenient there for the driver!

Baby should not be wrapped or swaddled when put into the capsule or carseat. The straps should be adjusted to hold baby in place, then a blanket can be tucked over baby for warmth if needed.

The most important job to be done well before baby is due to be born is to have baby's capsule or carseat correctly installed in your car. Whether you use a baby capsule or a car seat, it is essential to follow the manufacturer's recommendations about installation especially which way to face the capsule or carseat for newborns. It is also wise to have the installation done by an expert car seat fitter, or checked by one if you have done it yourself. Do not leave this job until after baby is born. Many parents have been caught out because baby came along earlier than expected and had to get the installation done in a hurry. If buying a second-hand car seat or capsule be sure to examine all the straps and fittings to ensure there is no damage or wear which could make it unsafe for re-use, and check it conforms to current recommendations and standards.

BABY'S PRAM / STROLLER

MOST PARENTS FIND their pram becomes their longest serving piece of baby equipment. It is a major purchase so deserves some thought and research as there is a staggering range of choices on display in the baby shops and on-line.

It is important to consider how you are likely to use your pram. Will you need to walk to go shopping, or are you more likely to take it in your car to the shopping centre? How big is your car boot, and how small does the pram fold down? How easy is it to fold down, and up, and how heavy is it to lift to put into the car? Will you use it inside the house for settling baby or moving baby around the house with you during his sleep times? Do the wheels get caught on furniture when manoeuvring in smaller spaces? Are the handles convertible from front facing, to back facing? When your baby is small you'll want to be able to look into the pram as you are walking along, and to easily attend to baby as needed. As baby gets older he will prefer to face the way you are going so he can see the world. Some prams allow for both options and others don't.

I suggest you go to the baby shops and test drive them first. Don't try them out empty, put some shopping into the demo models so you can compare how they handle with some weight. Check whether they might easily tip backwards if a heavy nappy bag is placed on the handles. Try out the brakes – how easy are they to put on and take off? Ask other parents about the features they do and don't like about their prams. When you have decided on your preferred model and features, check the prices on-line. You may find it on sale or maybe second hand. If someone has offered to buy your pram for you make sure you are closely involved in the selection process. For a detailed description of the many different types of prams strollers and joggers visit: **www.birth.com.au/Baby-products**

FEEDING REQUIREMENTS

IF YOU ARE PLANNING TO breast feed your baby all you need to buy are two or three comfortable, well-fitting maternity bra's and a packet of breast pads. It is a good idea to buy one bra that is a size bigger than you expect as in the first week or two of lactation most women are astonished at how big their breasts become. They settle down after a few weeks, so don't spend a lot on the biggest bra, just make sure you have one for when you need it.

Unless you are having twins **you do not need a breastfeeding pillow**. Watch the **video "How to Breastfeed your Baby"** which demonstrates optimal positioning and attachment. A few cushions for Mother's comfortable support when breastfeeding will be helpful, however a breastfeeding pillow can obstruct baby's instinctive preference to be in close body contact and positioned facing the mother.

If you have concerns about your breasts or nipples discuss them with your Midwife or a Lactation Consultant before purchasing any of the many 'aids' which are on the market. You will probably need a breast pump if your baby is born prematurely, or if you encounter problems with your milk supply – too little or too much. Whether using a hand or electric pump it is essential that the flange size is correct for your nipples. Nipple Shields also should be correctly sized to suit the mother's nipple, not the size of the baby's mouth.

Dummies or pacifiers and bottle feeding with a teat are not recommended for breastfeeding babies because they alter the way baby uses his tongue, which can confound baby's tongue action when breastfeeding. If you choose to have a dummy on hand, choose one with a round bulb end (cherry style). The "orthodontic" or flat/wedge shaped dummies encourage a sucking action which makes the back of the tongue "hump" which can be detrimental to baby's suckling action at the breast.

If you are planning to bottle feed your baby with formula you will need to take a tin of formula with you to hospital, and two bottles with teats will be ample. Formula is always made up just before it is to be given to baby so only one bottle will be in use at a time. Which bottle and teat your baby prefers is a matter of trial and error, so avoid buying more than a couple of bottles until you have worked out which one suits your new baby. You will also need a bottle brush for cleaning, and if you wish to sterilise feeding items you will find a microwave steam steriliser is an easy and cheap option. Chemical sterilising solutions are no longer recommended.

BABY BATH

YOU CAN USE A BABY bath, or a clean basin, sink or laundry trough to bath your baby. Some baby baths come with a stand and an outlet hose to make emptying easier. You may be able to borrow a baby bath from a friend as they tend to be used for the first few months and then baby graduates to being bathed in the adult size bath. Placing a baby bath into your adult bath and using it there can make filling and emptying the baby bath easier. If Mum has had a caesarean section a full baby bath is too heavy for her to lift or carry. A baby bath thermometer is an inexpensive, handy and reassuring item to have for checking the bath water temperature which should be around 37C.

Baby does not need to be bathed every day – it can be an alternate-day job, and washing of face, hands and bottom (in that order) can be done instead if it's not convenient to do a bath. You can also take baby into the shower instead of bathing them in the traditional way – this is a good job for Dad but Mum needs to be on hand to take baby out to dry and dress him. There are no rules – do what works for you and find what your baby enjoys.

HANDY HINT - Keep a small bottle of olive oil with your baby bath equipment.

To remove dried blood from a newborn's scalp - a few drops of olive oil mixed with some baby bath solution in the palm of your hand, then gently rubbed on baby's head before a bath will cleanse it when rinsed without rubbing the delicate and possibly tender scalp. A few drops of olive oil in the bath water moisturises baby's skin without coating or clogging pores.

BABY SWINGS AND SEATS

MANY LITTLE SEATS AND bouncers of all descriptions are available and are fairly inexpensive. These are handy for placing baby between phases of a feed, or until baby shows tired signs and is ready to be swaddled and settled in bed to sleep. For safety reasons it is very important that they are always used on the floor and are not placed on a bench or table. They are outgrown quite quickly and are often an item which a friend is happy to loan you.

Although these are not essential many parents find a simple mesh bouncer or mechanised baby swing is very helpful for unsettled babies. Bouncers or swings are a handy way to have baby nearby allowing some 'hands free' time for parents to get some other tasks done in the early months. Young babies tend to enjoy the swings for short periods only, and a swing can be helpful to sooth a tired baby. Many swings have music and mobile options, and can swing front to back or side to side. It's good to try before you buy, so borrow one if possible in case your baby does not like swinging or rocking. Avoid baby sleeping in rockers - baby should be laid flat in a bassinet, cot or baby bed to sleep safely. Avoid beanbag style and soft filled pillow type sleepers which do not comply with safe sleep recommendations.

BABY SLINGS & CARRIERS

SLINGS OR CARRIERS CAN BE really helpful when baby needs to be close to you and you need to have your hands free. Make sure the carrier provides you with lower back support. Some carriers have a newborn insert option allowing it to be used from the early days through to toddling.

There are many variations and styles of slings. If possible, borrow a few different types of slings and try them out after baby is born so you can buy the type that you find most comfortable when you know what you need, or don't need.

PLAYMATS AND ENTERTAINMENT CENTRES

A LITTLE TIME ON THE floor is a good thing; babies benefit developmentally if they are not "packaged" upright in a seat of some kind all the time. However, newborn babies do not need entertaining with lots of gadgets and toys. It is far better for young babies to be 'entertained' by interacting with a friendly human face which enhances baby's interest in communication, and sense of security and belonging. Too many toys or noises can be overwhelming for a newborn, so again – less is more. **Topic 9 – Fun Times** provides information about your baby's socialisation milestones and best forms of entertainment.

SOME EXTRA ADVICE FROM AN EXPERIENCED MUM

Handling your baby safely will be much easier if your fingernails are SHORT! Long fingernails present a real hazard each time you need to latch and detach baby during breastfeeding or calm baby by allowing him to suck your finger. You risk scratching baby's delicate skin every time you dress and undress baby and change baby's nappy for the ump-teenth time. Long fingernails are also harder to keep clean and can harbour dangerous germs.

A TIP FROM AN EXPERIENCED DAD

When friends ask what is your baby's due date – add a week!

This will save you the hassle of being pestered by "interested others" if and when your due date goes past without baby arriving.

DID YOU KNOW? Kissing your baby changes your breast milk. Did you know that the undeniable urge to cover your baby in kisses serves a biological purpose? When a mother kisses her baby, she samples the pathogens on baby's face, which then travel to mum's lymphatic system. Mum's body then creates antibodies to fight those pathogens, which baby receives through breast milk.

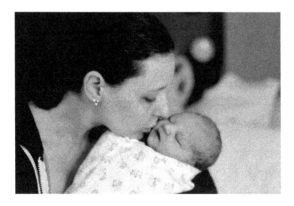

References: Lauren Sompayrac, author of *How The Immune Systems Works*, 2011. Wiley-Blackall

TOPIC 2
Early Decisions

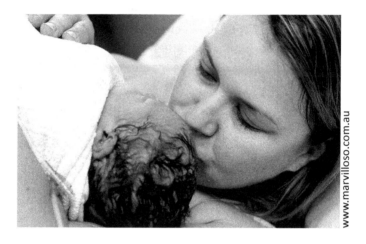

www.marvilloso.com.au

THERE ARE A FEW IMPORTANT THINGS you will need to consider before baby is born, or soon afterwards. Welcome to parenthood and the long, long road of making decisions on behalf of your child!

CORD CLAMPING

DURING YOUR ANTENATAL visits you are likely to be asked about your preferences for labour and birth. A commonly overlooked part of the Birth Plan is the management of the third stage of labour, particularly regarding clamping and cutting of the baby's umbilical cord. When the question of who will cut the baby's cord is discussed it is also important to consider the benefits for baby of **delayed cord** clamping.

For many birth attendants *immediate* cord clamping is their standard practise and you may need to specifically request to have delayed cord clamping if that is your preference. The blood in the cord and the placenta is part of baby's blood supply, and research has shown immediate cord clamping and cutting deprives the baby of about 50mls of his blood volume. Delayed cord clamping, even 30 seconds delay, has been shown to benefit the baby's lungs by maximising his circulating blood volume as he makes the transition to breathing for himself. **The main benefits of delayed cord clamping are:**

- The intact umbilical cord provides a "lifeline" to the baby, and continues to pulsate after the birth providing him/her with oxygen-rich blood from the placenta while he/she begins to breathe. Baby is therefore less likely to need resuscitation after birth, or to experience respiratory distress.
- Delayed cord clamping allows the baby to receive his/her full blood volume and optimal iron stores, reducing the likelihood of baby developing anaemia in infancy.
- The placenta is less bulky making it more readily expelled by the mother.
- Keeping the cord intact ensures the newborn stays close to his/her mother, helping to initiate bonding and breastfeeding, and reducing stress.

Visit: **www.birthjourney.com** for more information about physiological management of the third stage of labour.

If you are considering CORD BLOOD COLLECTION for long term storage, understand that this process deprives your baby of 100 to 200mls of his blood volume at a critical time of his life. Parents considering "banking" their baby's cord blood need to carefully weigh up the benefits for baby of having his full circulating blood volume intact (when he actually needs it) against the likelihood of "needing" that stored cord blood in many years' time.

VITAMIN K

VITAMIN K (K1:PHYLLOQUINONE) given at birth can prevent a **very rare** but often fatal bleeding disorder of babies called **Vitamin K Deficiency Bleeding of the newborn (VKDB)**. When this disorder occurs in older babies it is called Late Onset Vitamin K Deficiency Bleeding. It is routine practise in Australia to give all newborn babies Vitamin K, usually by intramuscular injection shortly after their birth.

The dose given by injection is 20,000 times the dose needed to protect the baby. The risk of VKDB in babies who have not had Vitamin K is 0.25-1.7 cases per 100 births, so most babies who receive Vitamin K do not actually need it.

Certain babies are at higher risk of VKDB. Babies born prematurely or very small, babies needing surgery and those who experience traumatic births resulting in bruises are more vulnerable. These babies should always be given Vitamin K by injection. Babies born to mothers who are taking anticonvulsant medications, anti-tubercular drugs, and Vitamin K antagonists (eg. Warfarin) during pregnancy are at greater risk of VKDB. These mothers may be given Vitamin K treatment in the last few weeks of their pregnancy to reduce their baby's risk of VKDB after birth.

ORAL VITAMIN K is an alternative to the intramuscular injection. In Australia the same product is used for oral administration as is used for intramuscular injection, however an oral version is available in other countries. When vitamin K is given orally according to the instructions it is just as effective as the injection. All three oral doses must be given – usually on the day of birth, between the third and fifth day, and at four weeks old. Oral Vitamin K spares the baby the painful experience of an injection at birth, and it is rapidly absorbed orally.

Well babies naturally begin to make their own vitamin K (K2:Menquinone) in their gastrointestinal tract from about 5 days onwards. Vitamin K is a fat soluble substance which occurs in higher volumes in colostrum and hindmilk, than in the foremilk. Breastfeeding mothers can also increase the amounts of vitamin K in their breastmilk by taking supplementary Vitamin K and including Vitamin K1-rich foods in their diet such as green leafy vegetables, vegetable oils, and dairy products.

Babies who are formula-fed receive additional amounts of vitamin K and actually do not need Vitamin K supplementation at birth, although they are almost always given Vitamin K by injection anyway.

Late onset VKDB is defined as unexpected bleeding in infants from 2-12 weeks of age. The incidence of this rare disorder is from 4.4 to 7.2 per 100,000 births, and may occur in breastfed babies who have had no Vitamin K supplementation, and babies who have intestinal malabsorption defects such as cholestatic jaundice and cystic fibrosis. If late onset VKDB occurs more than half of those affected babies will have acute intracranial (brain) haemorrhages.

If parents decide to decline giving their baby Vitamin K at birth they should be watchful for any signs of abnormal bleeding (from the nose, umbilicus, rectum or vomited blood), or on the skin as bruises appearing on the baby. Any signs of bleeding must be investigated immediately. Jaundice (yellow colouring of the skin or whites of the eyes) occurring after the first three weeks of life is not normal and a doctor should be consulted immediately if this happens. Ultimately it is the parents' decision whether to give Vitamin K by injection or orally, or not at all and you will be asked to sign a consent for one of these three options prior to having your baby in hospital.

Dr Sara Wickham has researched the topic of Vitamin K for newborns extensively. Here is some of her reliable advice:
"As with many birth and parenting decisions, it's not always an "all or nothing" decision. For instance: You may decide to have oral vitamin K rather than the injection. In this situation, be aware that Vitamin K is fat soluble. So in order to be properly absorbed by the baby's body, it should be given with or just after a feed. Also be aware that it tastes bitter. Many babies will try to spit out again and you might want to have your finger ready to scoot it back in! You may decide to wait and see and make a decision according to your situation. There are a few key information issues to consider. If your baby is breastfed and is slow to feed or has feeding problems, the chance of VKDB is higher and you may want to reconsider. If you or your baby have had antibiotics, this can increase the chance of VKDB. Again, you may want to take that into account. Likewise if your baby has a procedure such as a tongue tie division or circumcision".
Source: **https://sarawickham.com/articles-2/information-about-vitamin-k/**

HEPATITIS B VACCINATION

ANOTHER DECISION YOU WILL BE ASKED to make before or shortly after baby is born is whether to allow baby to be given a Hepatitis B Vaccination in the first few days of life. Hepatitis B is a viral infection which can cause short or long term liver disease. Carriers of the virus are able to pass the virus on to others. About one person in every 100 is a Hep B carrier in Australia.

Hepatitis B virus is found in infected body fluids including blood, vaginal secretions, semen and saliva, and can be transmitted by sexual contact, and contact with infected blood from cuts or sores, sharing razors, needles and syringes, needle stick injuries and body piercing. It can also be transmitted by sharing toothbrushes with an infected person or carrier, and babies may contract the virus from the blood of their infected mother during the birth process or if there is blood present in her breast milk. It is safe for a Hepatitis B positive mother to breastfeed her baby **if there is no blood in her milk or bleeding injuries to her nipples.**

Health Authorities in Australia recommend all babies be offered Hepatitis B Vaccination at birth, which is the first of a series of four injections given again at 2 months, 4 months and 6 months. Some babies are at high risk of being exposed to Hepatitis B, for example if either of the parents are Hepatitis B carriers or either of them has a past history of intravenous drug use, if they are likely to be living in an area where Hepatitis B infection is very high, or if the baby is likely to be cared for in a shared facility such as Day Care in the first 2 months of his life. Babies exposed to any of these risk factors should certainly be given the birth dose of Hep B vaccine.

Alternatively, if parents decide they do not fall into any of the above risk groups they can decline the birth dose of Hep B vaccine for their baby, and obtain it when the baby commences the routine vaccination program offered throughout Australia at 2 months of age. Three or more doses are required to be fully immunised, so if a baby does not have the first Hep B dose at birth would he would receive Hepatitis B vaccine at 2 months, 4 months and 12 months of age instead. It is every parent's responsibility to carefully examine their options regarding vaccinating their child, and their choices should be respected.

NEONATAL SCREENING TEST (NNST) OR 'HEEL PRICK' TEST

ALL BABIES IN AUSTRALIA are offered free screening for a number of hereditary disorders which are detected from a blood sample taken from the baby's heel after he is 48 hours old. All of the disorders are treatable, but if left undetected result in bad outcomes for the baby. The blood is collected on a special absorbent paper card, filling 3 little circles of blood which is sent away by the hospital or Midwife for testing. No news is good news – most people never have to think about it again. If an abnormality is found the parents are contacted quickly.

The procedure can fill parents with dread, but it can be conducted with minimal trauma for baby and the parents if the following things are done. Warm the baby's foot first – an easy way is to half-fill a disposable glove with warm water, tie a knot in the top and wrap the warm glove around the baby's foot for a few minutes before the Midwife starts the procedure. *(Some hospitals may have protocols which prohibit the midwife preparing baby's foot with warmth, however the parents can choose to carefully do this themselves). The baby will hardly notice the heel prick if he is breastfeeding first, so ask the Midwife to collect the blood while a breastfeed is in progress. Baby may squeal when the prick is done but can be immediately soothed by latching back on the breast, and will then probably feed happily throughout the blood collection process. If the Midwife refuses to do it that way you can ask for another Midwife who will perform the test that way. The NNST does not need to be traumatic for baby or the parents. The method of collecting blood with baby's leg held upwards and baby screaming throughout the procedure is outdated practise. For peace of mind it really is worth having this test done, especially if you ensure it is done with a minimum of drama or fuss.

HEARING SCREEN TEST

THIS IS ANOTHER CONSENT FORM for you to fill in! The hearing screen test is done when baby is quiet or asleep and the procedure does not hurt baby in any way. About one or two babies out every 1000 are born with significant hearing loss, and early detection results in early intervention and best outcomes. Healthy hearing is essential for baby's optimal development.

The test is conducted by a trained person using a special program on a laptop computer. Small pads are placed on baby's head and an earphone is placed over baby's ears – one at a time – delivering soft clicking sounds and the pads record baby's responses. The test usually only takes about ten minutes. If any problems are found further testing will be organised.

CIRCUMCISION

ALTHOUGH THIS IS NOT A SUBJECT that is likely to be raised by caregivers during pregnancy or soon after baby is born, some parents may be considering this option for their baby boy.   Circumcision of baby boys is no longer endorsed by most health professionals due to the risks of bleeding and infection, and the unnecessary pain experienced by the baby.   **No medical organisation in the world recommends routine circumcision of boys**. The Royal Australian College of Physicians, the British Medical Association and the American Academy of Paediatrics have issued position statements against male circumcision without medical reason.

Female circumcision is regarded as genital mutilation and circumcision of baby boys is the same. Baby boys experience excruciating pain during circumcision and for weeks afterwards, and can show behavioural changes such as frequent crying, avoidance of physical contact, reduced feeding and sleep disturbance following the procedure. Local anaesthetic creams do not provide adequate anaesthesia for the operation and a general anaesthetic poses significant risk for infants under the age of 6 months.

The most common reason I hear from parents wishing to have their baby boy circumcised is so his penis will look the same as his circumcised father's penis. However from a child's perspective, all adult male genitalia looks different to their own. The presence of pubic hair is a very obvious difference which children readily accept is "just how grown-ups look".

Little boys are fascinated with their own and other little boys' anatomy and function. They are very likely to question why a boy's circumcised penis looks so different to an intact boy's penis. A little boy is likely to have problems reasoning why his parents allowed part of his penis to be cut off when he was a baby, but he will readily accept that his circumcised father's glans is visible all the time rather than only sometimes when the foreskin is retracted.

Another common reason parents choose to have their sons circumcised is a belief that it is more hygienic. The hygiene habits of our modern society and bathing facilities are vastly different to those experienced by those from previous generations. Daily showering and hot running water (in indoor bathrooms) were not the norm as they are these days. Daily bathing provides adequate cleanliness in most developed world settings and hygiene care of baby boys and girls does not differ.

Circumcision does not reduce the risks of cancer of the penis or cervix. The risk factors for these cancers are cigarette smoking, and exposure to multiple strains of the human papilloma or wart virus (HPV) through unprotected sex with multiple partners. Penile cancer is extremely rare (1 in 100,000 men), and penile cancer can develop on the circumcision scar. Studies in industrialised nations such as Australia find that circumcision does not reduce the risk of transmission of sexually transmitted diseases.

Circumcision is unnecessary cosmetic surgery which carries significant risks. During the decision making process an important point for parents to consider is that it is a woman's right to choose in matters concerning her own body, and it should be a man's right to choose also. The appearance of the penis is a matter personal preference and only the owner of the penis has the right to decide about alterations to its appearance, structure and function. For more information visit: **www.birthjourney.com**

DO I WANT TO BREASTFEED OR BOTTLE FEED MY BABY?

THIS IS A QUESTION EVERY WOMAN should really consider carefully. Most pregnant women will already have encountered advice from well-meaning friends and family about how to best-feed their baby. Women may feel pressured to breastfeed their baby, even if it is not something that they feel comfortable about for a variety of reasons. Some women have doubts about their ability to breastfeed because their mother could not breastfeed them. The circumstances of a previous generation's experience of breastfeeding is unlikely to be relevant, unless a physical characteristic such as insufficient glandular tissue (IGT) has been inherited, and even then support strategies and understanding of IGT are vastly improved now.

 Women who have had breast surgeries (breast reduction, breast implants, nipple surgery) should seek advice from an International Board Certified Lactation Consultant (IBCLC) about their particular situation regarding breastfeeding as their expectations may not be accurate. These mothers-to-be may face difficulties establishing breastfeeding and expert advice provided BEFORE baby is born will guide them towards achieving their goals. For first-time Mums this is uncharted territory and a woman can't really know how she will feel about breastfeeding until she actually experiences it. Ultimately it is a personal decision only the mother can make about her body and her baby, and her decision should be respected and supported. Information about bottle feeding your baby is provided in **Topic 4 – Feedtime**.

Breastfeeding provides many benefits for baby. The first milk called colostrum is nutrient rich and is essential for establishing the baby's immune system in the gastrointestinal tract by providing "an abundance of bioactive factors which support and enhance the immunologic system of the newborn" (1). "Gut health" has become recognised as an essential component of overall lifelong wellbeing. **Breastmilk provides the optimal microbiome in the infant gastrointestinal tract for both protection and nutrition.** Breastfed babies experience fewer infections of the ears, chest, urinary tract and gastrointestinal tract. Breastfed babies have a reduced incidence of allergies such as asthma, eczema and coeliac and bowel disease, and reduced likelihood of obesity. Breastfed babies have reduced chance of developing diabetes and childhood cancers such as leukaemia. They have better eyesight, speech, dental development and have higher intelligence. Who wouldn't want all those benefits for their baby?

For Mothers breastfeeding reduces the risk of breast and ovarian cancer, osteoporosis, and they lose weight after the birth more easily than mothers who bottle feed their babies. The big winner for parents is the fact that breastmilk is free! It can cost around $2000 to formula feed a baby for one year. Formula-fed babies are 5 times more likely to be admitted to hospital with gastro-enteritis, and twice as likely to suffer from respiratory and ear infections. Babies fed formula are 5 times more likely to develop a urinary tract infection (UTI) and twice as likely to develop eczema or a wheeze if there is a family history of these problems.

Statistics in Australia indicate most Mothers begin their baby's life breastfeeding probably for all the above reasons. Unfortunately many women find developing the new skill of breastfeeding a real challenge if they encounter problems in

Reference: **https://www.ncbi.nlm.nih.gov/pmc/articles/PMC4414019/**

the early days and weeks. This can result in partial or full abandonment of breastfeeding even though they desperately wanted to succeed. The best way to ensure your baby gets the best start in life is to contact an International Board Certified Lactation Consultant well BEFORE your baby is due to be born, in order to receive pre-birth education and preparation for your breastfeeding experience.

ANTENATAL EXPRESSION OF COLOSTRUM

EXPRESSING AND COLLECTING colostrum from the breasts from 36 weeks of pregnancy has become a common recommendation for women who are planning to breastfeed. This may be particularly important for women who have gestational diabetes, or if a preterm birth is expected, eg twins. The DAME trial confirmed women with diabetes and a low risk pregnancy can safely express breastmilk in late pregnancy without causing harm to their babies and, for some first-time mothers, their babies will be less likely to receive formula in the first 24 hours of life if they have brought some colostrum with them to hospital.

In the DAME trial the median (total) amount of colostrum collected per woman was 5mls. Some pregnant women will harvest more, and others less, or none. The volumes of colostrum collected before baby is born does not necessarily represent the volumes of breastmilk a mother can expect to make after birth.

Watch this video which I present to learn how to express colostrum during pregnancy:

https://vimeo.com/420895736

Read this Australian Breastfeeding Association document for more information: **https://www.breastfeeding.asn.au/bfinfo/antenatal-expression-colostrum**. (Includes reference for the DAME trial).

TOPIC 3
Your First Days at Home

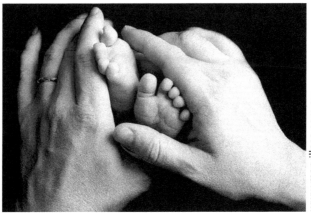

www.marvilloso.com.au

ALL NEW PARENTS WALK OUT of the hospital with their newborn feeling a mix of delight and anticipation about what lies ahead of them. I am sure every one of them hopes to do everything right, but knows they are bound to feel uncertain about what is going on with this new, utterly dependent little person they have created.

Even before leaving hospital both parents are likely to feel quite overwhelmed by their birthjourney and the experience of finally holding their baby in their arms. Especially for the Mother the excitement of the birth and responses of family and friends may make it difficult to rest, and the baby's need for frequent feeds and cuddles around the clock can result in absolutely exhausted parents heading out of the hospital car park with their precious cargo strapped into his baby capsule.

These early weeks at home with your new baby provide a precious time for parents and baby to bond as a family – this is your **Babymoon**. Cuddle baby skin to skin with Mum and with Dad often. This will enhance the hormones of love which enable bonding, and also comforts baby especially if she is unsettled or overtired. Rest together, and allow yourselves to have private quiet times enjoying and exploring your new life as parents.

You will cope best if you embrace the concept of your life following a 24 hour cycle for the first few months, and let go of "day and night" expectations. Understanding and accepting that this pattern is part of the new parent deal will help you to go with the flow of getting up in the night and permitting yourself to sleep in the daytime when you need to do so. This can be a real struggle for women who are used to being highly organised with everything in order. Exhaustion and sleep deprivation are a high price to pay for a tidy house.

SOME DO'S and SOME DON'T's

DO ACCEPT HELP. Pre-arrange it if you can by having a close family member who is experienced with new babies stay with you for a few days. Their job is to look after both the parents, so the parents can look after the baby. Cooking meals, shopping and intercepting unwanted phone calls and visitors are the main tasks of this helper. Moral support, reassurance and TLC will also help the new parents to adjust to the demands of their new roles.

DO get organised in the home before baby comes home. Make sure the home is clean and comfortable, and cupboards are well stocked with basic food (milk, bread, fruit and veges) and grocery items (nappies, toilet paper, sanitary pads, paracetamol). Have some cooked meals in the freezer ready to enjoy with a minimum of preparation, and accept offers of prepared meals from kind neighbours, friends and family. Eat nutritious meals and snacks and avoid take-aways.

DON'T allow visitors to come unless the time suits you. Yes, they are excited about the new baby and want to welcome him, but 'entertaining' can take up valuable rest times for the Mother in the daytime, and result in overtired parents and a fractious baby later. Work out a day and time for visitors – limit it to an hour or two maximum, and if they can't fit in with your plans they can come another day.   If they really care about you they will understand. If your friends want to bring you a meal or help with your washing – let them!

One subtle strategy to manage visitors who stay too long is to withdraw to your bedroom to rest or feed your baby. As long as you are in your living areas visitors will feel welcome. If they enter your bedroom most people will feel less comfortable in this more private zone of your home, and are more likely to realise it is time for them to leave.

DO have a sign ready to put on your front door – *"Mother and Baby sleeping – please do not disturb"* – and use it.

DO get out of doors and do some gentle exercise each day. A short walk to a park or around your own garden will help you to relax and enjoy nature and the outside world which will clear your head and lift your spirits if you are feeling like life has become a perpetual cycle of baby care. Plan a walk with baby in the pram or sling in the late afternoon which is a common time for babies to be unsettled.

DO any shopping that is absolutely necessary early in the day. Make the trips short, and if baby is coming with you be sure to take a well stocked nappy bag and be prepared to feed baby even if you plan to be back before feed time is expected. Babies don't read shopping or 'to do' lists.

DO keep your plans for each day really simple and focussed on your baby's needs. This is not the time to try to write that novel or PhD because you are home and expected to have so much spare time on your hands!

DO try to have your morning shower early – well, before lunchtime anyway.

DO sleep when your baby sleeps. You never know what kind of night you will have, so in the early days grab sleep whenever you can. Remember to put the sign on the door and the phone on silent.

Do prepare you pets for baby's arrival into their domain. Cats and dogs will be curious at least, and potentially jealous of the attention baby will inevitably demand and receive. It can be a confusing and confronting time for a pet which has enjoyed your full attention in the past.

One strategy which can be helpful – especially for dogs – is to take an old tea towel or clothing item like a T-shirt with you to the hospital, and place it inside baby's wraps so it gets baby's scent on it. When the item is taken home the pet can then be introduced to baby's scent without baby being present. Allow the pet to keep it, sleep on it, bury it or whatever he likes to make it familiar. Most pets will accept the baby more readily if they have been 'introduced' this way, prior to baby arriving in the home.

Try to maintain the pet's usual routines such as feed times and walks. Arrange for a friend or neighbour to walk your dog regularly if you are unable to manage this yourself. If you plan to make changes to the pet's sleep arrangements, do it well before baby is due so the pet is accustomed to their environmental changes well in advance.

SURVIVAL STRATEGIES

WHAT'S ALL THIS FUSS ABOUT SLEEP - Babies sleep a lot anyway – don't they?

Do you need the same amount of sleep as your partner, your friend, your mother or your sister? Probably not, because each individual's sleep requirements differ according to lifestyle, age and personal preferences. Babies' sleep requirements vary too, and realising this fact will save some parents untold anguish as they reconcile their expectations about their baby's sleep patterns with their new parent reality.

Newborn babies need to feed frequently – 8 to 12 times in every 24 hours. Each feed may take an hour or more, including nappy changes, burps and cuddles. This means the potential time for sleep between feeds for baby and parents is limited to snatches of an hour or two at best, and this is what parents should expect. Most babies will naturally pop in a longer sleep time of 2 to 4 hours somewhere in each 24 hour day which parents will truly appreciate especially if they also manage to sleep at the same time as baby. It is common for babies to "cluster feed" - feeding every 30-60 minutes or so for a period of the day – typically in the late afternoon or early evening. Be prepared to go to bed early as many young babies have their longest sleep between 8pm and midnight.

You may ask *"How long does this go on, and how do parents with a new baby survive?"* Take heart, the most demanding period of sleep deprivation is usually the first four to eight weeks of baby's life. Imposing a 'routine' on a baby is potentially harmful to baby's physical and mental growth and development. It is normal and necessary for baby to feed regularly day and night for the first few months to nurture his growing body and brain, and this is nature's way of establishing and maintaining Mother's milk supply. Baby will change his sleep and feed patterns as he grows and it is important to 'go with the flow' as he develops. Following you baby's cues and responding to his needs promptly makes for a contented baby and a relaxed family life.

Here are a few strategies which can help the new family to adapt to life together, and enhance the enjoyment of having a baby in the house.

Learn to observe when baby is tiring, such as fussing, yawning, making 'jerky' movements, and offer sleep strategies before he progresses to crying. Offering the breast again to suckle to sleep is physiologically normal, and usually effective. (This is a breastfeeding mother's superpower!)

Swaddling baby comfortably but firmly in a soft wrap will help baby feel secure, and also reduce self-disturbance due to the 'startle reflex' which all young babies demonstrate when awake and asleep. **Watch the New Baby 101 video demonstrating how to swaddle baby** "How to Swaddle Your Baby"

Warming baby's bedding before putting him in, and resting your hands gently on him for a few minutes after laying him down may also assist baby to relax and drift off to sleep. (*Never leave a heat pack or hot water bottle in the bed with baby).

If the time between feeds extends beyond four hours during the day, and it suits you, gently unwrap baby and waken her for feeding. If she has had frequent feeds during the daytime she might have a longer sleep period sometime during the night. Bliss!

Getting advice - there is bound to be lots of advice coming your way from well-meaning friends and relatives which may be helpful, or sometimes confronting. Seek help from health professionals such as your Midwife or Child Health Nurse to talk over any struggles and concerns, or if feeding is not going well contact a Certified Lactation Consultant for advice **http://www. LCANZ.com.au   https://ilca.org/why-ibclc-falc/**

If you seek information on the internet ensure it is from reliable health professionals, and avoid forums and information from unqualified sources. In particular there is some potentially dangerous advice about structured feeding and sleep routines for babies which have become popular among some parents. Midwives, Lactation Consultants and Paediatricians warn against forcing babies, especially newborns, to 'fit into' structured routines because it is dangerous to baby's physical and mental health if his basic needs are not met promptly by responsive parents.

 Be discerning; believe in and trust your instincts – you know your baby better than anyone else, so if a suggestion doesn't feel right to you, it probably isn't! You will develop your own parenting style which is right for you and your baby. For excellent parenting support visit Pinky's Blog **www.pinkymckay. com.au** and link into her free email support systems.

Handy Tip for hungry, time-poor parents

PRE-PACKAGED MEALS ARE GENERALLY regarded as inferior from a taste perspective, however it is better for busy new parents to eat a well-balanced packaged frozen meal than expensive and calorie overloaded take-aways. **Lite N Easy** frozen meals are nutritious, tasty and satisfying and are delivered to your door. A selection of your chosen favourites will be a welcome find in your freezer when you don't have the time or energy to shop or cook. **www. liteneasy.com.au**

TOPIC 4
Feedtime (Part 1)

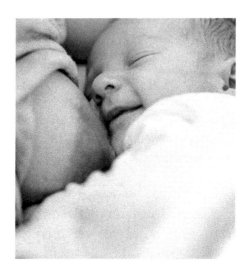

THE VAST MAJORITY OF QUESTIONS which new parents have relate to feeding their newborn baby.   Consequently this topic has been divided into two parts – Part 1 – Feedtime – Understanding Baby's Needs and Part 2 – Feedtime – Concerns and Problems.   All the basic information parents need about feeding their baby is covered in these two topics.   The focus is on questions relating to the BABY, however essential breastfeeding information is included to assist the mother to develop her own personal breastfeeding style, which also suits her baby.

PREPARING FOR BREASTFEEDING

If you are planning to breastfeed your baby, the best advice I can give you is to **prepare in advance of your birth** by attending a breastfeeding education session with a midwife or lactation consultant. First-time mothers naturally focus on preparing for the birth of their baby and often underestimate how demanding learning to breastfeed can be, and how helpful a good understanding of the basics will be when her baby is in her arms, and hungry!

Pre-birth breastfeeding education via reputable on-line services or books will prove to be a valuable investment. Booking a pre-birth education session with an International Board Certified Lactation Consultant will provide insight about physical features of the mother-to-be's breasts and any relevant medical history to consider regarding preparing for breastfeeding, as well as learning hand expression of colostrum and basic positioning and attachment techniques.

UNDERSTANDING BABY'S NEEDS

BABIES KNOW *HOW* to feed and they know *when* they need to feed, and they give clear signals to let their carers know their needs – these are called **Feeding Cues.** These cues or signals progressively intensify as baby's need to be fed increases.

Early cues include stirring from sleep and stretching, opening the mouth and licking lips. The baby may progress to turning his head, increasing his physical movements, and putting his hands to his mouth. Baby may mouth around, seeking the breast. **Late cues** include agitated body movements, crying and becoming upset and red in the face. If baby becomes upset and cries you need to CALM baby down before you commence a breastfeed. Attaching a crying baby to the breast will result in a poor latch and potentially injure mother's nipple – no fun for anyone! Calm baby down by cuddling, putting baby skin to skin on Mum's chest, talking gently to baby and stroking his head or back. A clean finger placed in baby's mouth, resting gently on the tongue will coax baby to suck the finger and calm down.

The important message here is – respond to your baby's **EARLY cues** as soon as possible after you see them. Regardless of whether you baby is being breastfed or bottle fed it is crucial to your baby's physical and mental wellbeing to respond to feeding cues promptly. Babies have small stomachs and efficient digestive systems, and they are in a persistent state of growth and development. They need to be fed frequently **day and night** to effectively sustain their rapidly growing bodies and brains. Unfortunately some parents do not realise how important this really is, and coax baby to wait a particular timeframe between feeds by using a dummy or other methods of delaying feeds. This is stressful for baby and detrimental to his health, and inevitably leads to other problems for baby.

Both breastfeeding and bottle feeding baby are covered in this book, with the focus on understanding normal feeding behaviours, and enabling feeding skills.

BREASTFEEDING BASICS

SOME WOMEN HAVE AN UNREALISTIC expectation that breastfeeding will "just happen" and may experience surprise, disappointment and frustration in the early hours and days of motherhood, finding breastfeeding just seems to be too hard! Breastfeeding is like learning to drive a car. It doesn't matter how much you **want** to drive a car, or how often you sit in the passenger seat carefully **watching** how to steer and change gears and use the clutch and the accelerator. Everyone learning to drive will bunny hop the car and grind the gears, and find the co-ordination of the pedals and the gears in combination with all other aspects of driving is a challenging new skill to master. Later it will all become 'second nature' and hardly require concentration to co-ordinate the actions at all, but in the beginning it requires effort and may involve some frustrations as co-ordination develops. Learning to breastfeed involves mastering a new set of co-ordination skills and it takes some time to gain confidence.

Breastfeeding is the culmination of the process of growing and giving birth to your baby. This extraordinary continuum has ensured the survival and development of our species. Modern women may doubt their own capacity to completely nurture their child but scientific discoveries continue to confirm the wondrous properties and unique benefits of human breast milk from newborn to toddlerhood and beyond.

HOW DOES THIS ALL HAPPEN?

MILK, IN THE FORM OF COLOSTRUM, is present from about the fourth month of pregnancy onwards. At birth, the delivery of the placenta triggers a reduction in the woman's progesterone levels that removes the inhibition of milk production and allows the elevated levels of prolactin to function.

Increased amounts of blood and lymph in the breast form the nutrients for milk production. These fluids cause the breasts to become fuller, heavier, and sometimes tender. As regular, frequent breastfeedings progress, this normal fullness diminishes. By about two weeks postpartum, when lactation is established, the breasts become comfortable soft and pliable, even when they are full with milk. Regular frequent feedings will maintain this condition (Lauwers & Swisher, 2005, p308).

Breastfeeding a Newborn Baby Be guided by your baby's cues as to when he wants to feed and for how long. During the first few days when baby's breastfeeds provide nutritious colostrum the feedings may be frequent and irregular in duration. Colostrum is highly concentrated, and baby's stomach capacity is small so the quantity of colostrum required to satisfy his needs is also small. Alternating sides each time the baby goes to the breast will stimulate the breasts, assisting the transition from colostrum to breast milk production (lactogenesis). Baby's stomach will gradually stretch in size as the volumes of colostrum and transitional milk progressively increase over the first 48 hours.

Feeding Frenzy Around day 2-3 baby often wants to feed more frequently, maybe 1-2 hourly. Baby has passed lots of black coloured meconium poos, emptying out his gastro-intestinal tract, and his stomach capacity is increasing in size in preparation for milk feeds. He's hungry! So feed him! This frequent feeding is nature's way of 'calling in the milk' and Mother's body will respond accordingly. Frequent breastfeeds in the early days has been shown to reduce the incidence of engorgement when the milk arrives. Skin-to-skin contact with baby, allowing baby to smell, hear and touch you and avoiding separations so you can respond to his feeding cues immediately will facilitate your 'milk coming in'.

The milk arrives Mother's breasts feel heavy, warm and may leak prior to or during feeds. Nature often overcompensates in the beginning, but it will settle down. Moist warm heat in the form of warm showers or warm wet cloths applied to the breasts will enhance 'letdown' to help the milk flow. Hand expressing a little milk before latching baby can relieve a tense areola and make it easier for baby to latch and feed effectively.

If the breasts are engorged and hot, applying cold treatments AFTER feeding from the breast (or expressing) can reduce inflammation and provide comfort. The easiest way to apply cold treatment is to soak a small towel with water, wring it out, fold it longways and place it flat in a freezer for a few minutes. The chilled towel can be wrapped around the engorged breast to aid vasoconstriction of the stretched breast tissue. Excessive use of cold treatments can reduce the flow of milk, so cease cold treatments once relief is gained, and only use it **after** milk has been removed by feeding or expressing.

Phases of a breastfeed When your milk first 'comes in' baby may be full and satisfied in one session or phase at the breast, as his stomach capacity has to stretch to accommodate the bigger volume of milk taken during the feed. Over the next day or so this will gradually change and baby will begin to seek a second session or phase of each feed, and sometimes, perhaps, a third!

Typically, baby will start the feed enthusiastically gulping down the fast-flowing milk from the full breast. This first phase of the feed may be completed in quite a short time, maybe 5-10 minutes. Baby will appear fully satisfied and will often drop off to sleep ("milk drunk"). The fast flowing milk baby has taken during this first phase of the feed is likely to be high in wonderful nutrients and fluid, but has very little fat content. Baby will sleep a short time – maybe 5- 30 minutes, and then stir. He has partially digested the milk taken in the first phase and now "cues" to continue the breastfeed.

Breast milk storage capacity varies greatly from woman to woman, and most breastfeeding women find one breast is more productive than the other – this is normal. Breast fullness also varies depending on whether feeding during the night or daytime. If the breast baby fed from previously still feels quite heavy with milk, it is advisable to **return the baby to the same breast** for the second phase of the feed. The milk he takes in the second phase of the feed is likely to now be milk which is higher in fat (however, this is not visible). This fattier milk will be digested more slowly than the milk taken earlier, and helps baby feel comfortable and satisfied. He may even repeat this a third or fourth time at some feeds. Be flexible about feeding and trust his cues.

At the next breastfeed you offer the opposite breast first, following the baby's cues as above.   This pattern ensures both breasts are well drained a number of times during each 24 hour period, enhancing the establishment of an ample breastmilk supply.   As baby grows he may drain the first breast in a couple of phases and still want more, so the feed may need to be completed on the second breast. In this case start the next feed on the breast which was drained the least – probably the second breast.

Women with smaller breastmilk storage capacity may need to feed baby from both breasts, sometimes several times, for baby to be satisfied. There are no rules, however returning baby to the starting breast at least once (if possible), before offering the second breast can ensure the breast is well drained and stimulates ample milk production. Women with smaller breasts still make ample volumes of milk – it is just received by baby in more phases as she switches sides more frequently. Baby will let her know when she has had enough.

Other terms used for this natural style of breastfeeding are "demand feeding" and "responsive feeding". This differs from "scheduled feeding" and is likely to result in somewhat irregular intervals between feeds, although feeding patterns will emerge. Each mother-baby combination is unique and responsive feeding ensures baby's individual and frequently changing needs are met optimally.

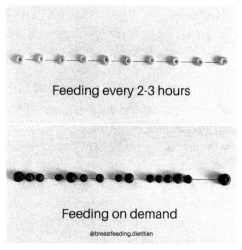

Feeding every 2-3 hours

Feeding on demand

@breastfeeding.dietitian

Source: Robyn Price
breastfeedingdietitian.com

So each breastfeed is usually comprised of a few instalments. Just as an adult varies the size of meals eaten according to hunger, and meals may be comprised of several courses, babies vary their feeds too. Young babies particularly need to take each 'meal' in a few stages, with rest times in between each stage to allow comfortable digestion.

Consider when you go out for a meal at a nice restaurant. You order your entree, and eat is quite quickly and enthusiastically because you were hungry! Some time goes by before your main course arrives. Your initial hunger is curbed so that's OK. Your main meal arrives and you steadily consume it, less quickly than the entree, but enjoying it just the same. You feel full. Nevertheless, you might still have a look at the dessert menu. OK, let's have dessert – you're ready for it by the time it arrives. Now you feel really satisfied and you relax into some after dinner conversation. A bit later you may want coffee and maybe after dinner mints too... but of course you don't do that every meal – just sometimes. The whole dinner process usually takes about an hour or so – reasonable and acceptable, right?

Isn't it reasonable and acceptable that a young baby's feed may be consumed over a similar timeframe and in several instalments if that is what baby demonstrates by his cues that is what he needs? Some feeds will be completed in less time and fewer instalments according to baby's hunger and thirst. Think of baby's breastfeed instalments like "Entrée, Main, Dessert". Be flexible, respond to your baby's early feeding cues and your baby will be contented and thrive, and hopefully sleep well between most feeds too.

In general, the baby's needs should determine feeding length. When the flow of milk diminishes from one breast, the sucking rate will move from the long, drawing nutritive suck to a faster, gentler suck. The baby's eyes will close, his fists will relax, and his hands will come away from his face. He may release the breast and let it slide out of his mouth. Allowing the baby to remove himself from the breast will ensure that he has received (sufficient milk) needed for optimal growth. Limiting the time spent on the breast may result in the baby receiving insufficient fatty milk. Flexibility on the mothers part will allow for variations in the baby's nursing style, hunger, and daily temperament (Lauwers & Swisher, 2005, p308).

Avoid giving bottle feeds to breastfed babies Many parents consider giving their newborn a bottle of expressed breastmilk to allow someone else, usually baby's father, the opportunity to feed the baby. Although this may seem an attractive idea especially if the mother imagines the bliss of sleeping through that feed time, it is not advisable for several reasons.

Introducing bottle feeds using a teat requires baby to suck very differently than how he does at the breast. The breastfeeding baby's tongue massages the breast tissue and the nipple which fills baby's mouth, working in union with the natural suck-swallow-breath rhythm that nature has designed to allow safe, comfortable feeding. Breastfeeding also enhances the development of the baby's oral and facial anatomy as he grows.

When a baby is given milk by a teat (which has holes in the tip) the milk pours straight into the mouth and throat, and baby responds by swallowing the milk. The rate of flow of milk dictates baby's suck-swallow-breath action, and often forces baby to feed faster and take greater volumes than is comfortable for baby. The tongue is shaped to conform to the teat and works in a piston-like action using the tongue muscles differently to when breastfeeding. This can quickly confound baby's natural and instinctive tongue action at the breast, and "derail" the baby from breastfeeding if she develops a "flow preference" for bottle feeding. Consequently it is not advisable to introduce a bottle and teat for feeds until baby is well established with breastfeeding, after about 6 weeks of age. (Detailed information about the "Paced Bottle Feeding" technique is provided in the Bottle Feeding section).

Another reason bottle feeds are not a good idea is the effect on the mother's breasts. If her breasts are not drained regularly (for example, if a breastfeed is missed) the breasts quickly become over-full and engorged, which can lead to problems such as blocked ducts and mastitis. **If baby is given a bottle feed the mother actually needs to be expressing her breasts at the same time to avoid these problems.** If the breasts are not drained well and frequently, the breasts' chemistry automatically changes to down-regulate her milk production, which will reduce the mother's milk supply. Breastfeeding baby directly is optimal for both mother and baby, and the partner can help more by doing nappy changes and cuddling baby to sleep, so Mum can get some rest after breastfeeding.

Just when you think you know what to expect – it changes!

Be prepared for your baby to change his pattern of feeding from time to time. This usually coincides with a "growth spurt or developmental leap" and baby will demand feeds more frequently for a day or two. To facilitate the process of increasing your supply you may need to abandon whatever plans you had for that day and 'just feed the baby'. If you've missed a lot of sleep overnight because of a feeding frenzy, go back to bed with your baby and feed him whenever he cues (or "on demand") and your body will respond by increasing your milk supply within 24-48 hours. These episodes of more frequent feeding are not only about adjusting the volume of milk produced, but also baby's changing nutritional needs. The constituents (recipe) of your breastmilk will also automatically change to suit your growing baby's needs. How this happens is still not fully understood, but nature provides perfectly for growing babies when mothers follow their baby's lead.

Giving supplementary feeds during this time will interfere with Mother's body's response to the delicate lactation process, so AVOID giving formula feeds unless absolutely necessary. Frequent drainage of the breasts, rest and good nutrition are key to natural breastmilk adjustments to meet your baby's growing needs – so look after yourself! Growth spurt feeding frenzies are fairly predictable in term babies, typically occurring at 2-3 days ("calling your milk in"); usually again around 2 or 3 weeks, again at around 6 weeks, very commonly around 3 months and again around 6 months of age. Interestingly, when breastfeeding women are having problems with perceived insufficient breastmilk supply and they review when the problem first arose, it often coincides with one of the typical growth/feeding frenzy stages – around 3 days, 3 weeks, 6 weeks, 3 or 6 months. If mothers are prepared to expect these changes to feeding behaviours they are more likely to cope with it appropriately and continue to successfully breastfeed their babies.

If baby is feeding frequently and well, gaining weight, has a normal output of 6 to 8 nappies with a minimum of 3 poos per day up until about 6 weeks of age, parents can be confident breastfeeding is going well.

HOW TO BREASTFEED YOUR BABY

EVERY MOTHER AND BABY combination is unique, and there is no single way to breastfeed that is right for everyone. Research into babies' instinctive feeding reflexes and behaviours has informed us over recent years. We now understand how these reflexes enable babies to feed in the most comfortable way for themselves and their mothers, and to optimise milk transfer in the process. I emphasise the following information is provided to guide the process of learning to breastfeed comfortably and successfully, and mothers can adapt their personal method to suit their own anatomy and their baby's individual preferences, which will change as they grow.

SKIN TO SKIN AND BREAST CRAWL

THIS IS THE STARTING POINT of the intimate relationship between mother and baby, but it is much more than a warm-fuzzy-feeling thing to do. Skin to skin contact with baby laid on mother's bare chest is the natural protective 'habitat' of the newborn baby, and this positioning switches on baby's brain to instinctively search for the breast. Baby begins by lifting his head, bobbing and stroking his face and cheeks on her skin, and with upper body movements and perhaps crawling motions of his legs and feet, he begins wriggling purposefully towards a breast. The mother instinctively gives baby gentle support of his body keeping him closely snuggled against her body. As his face touches the breast and his chin contacts the breast tissue under the nipple, he will gape his mouth widely with his tongue down, and "launch to latch" to the breast. In the seconds that follow baby's latch creates a vacuum as he draws breast tissue in to fill his mouth, and suckling begins.

This is an inborn ability that all <u>well</u> newborns can demonstrate when given the opportunity and right environment. In ideal circumstances for a well newborn baby and mother, baby can "self latch" following a breast crawl, or when being held with his face resting against the mother's breast. This is an awesome sight and experience when it happens! Even if the first hour after birth has been interrupted and baby has not breastfed in that time, recreating the skin to skin environment and supporting mother-baby natural interactions and responses may result in an unassisted latch and suckle. Midwives are experts at enabling mothers to breastfeed their newborn babies. It is essential, of course, that these early breastfeeds are comfortable for the mother too.

The advances of Biological Nurturing and baby-led, mother-guided approaches, recently referred to as the physiologic approaches to breastfeeding initiation, help empower both women...and are now widely applied in breastfeeding initiation. However, physiologic approaches are not enough to ensure successful breastfeeding for many women in the weeks and months post-birth.

In the early hours and days of life babies do best if they are cuddled frequently in skin to skin contact, and this will enhance the baby's instinctive responses and the mother's breastfeeding skill development. Beginning breastfeeds with a breast crawl will ensure baby is ready and natural feeding reflexes are 'switched on'.

Mother can help baby to attach to the breast however she finds works best for her baby and her own comfortable breastfeeding experience. **Watch the New Baby 101 video: "How to breastfeed your baby". https://www.youtube. com/watch?v=NTblsdJ_qck**

Note: The mother in the video uses her hand folded beside her areola to assist the baby to latch. She has found this is what works for her. Techniques such as gently shaping the breast or placing a finger or thumb above the nipple to tilt it upwards and into baby's mouth may also work well, provided her fingers are not placed anywhere that obstructs baby's face, chin and mouth contacting the breast.

POSITIONING BABY TO BREASTFEED

START BY UNWRAPPING YOUR BABY. His hands should be uncovered and free to move naturally to enable his instinctive seeking and feeding behaviours. Baby needs to be calm to breastfeed. The Mother can be sitting upright, or leaning back and comfortably supported if she prefers a more laid-back position. The mother's breast should be allowed to fall naturally; large breasted women may need to roll up a face washer or small towel and place it under the breast to support it if it is very heavy.

Baby's body needs to be turned to fully face the mother's body, and cuddled in close contact. The mother can hold and support baby over the back and shoulders, with baby's head unrestricted, allowing baby to tilt his head back as he approaches to breast. The Transition Hold (sometimes called cross-cradle hold) is often easiest for mothers to use to achieve a deep latch when learning to breastfeed a newborn baby, however the Cradle Hold can also work well if the mother's breasts and nipples are ideally shaped.

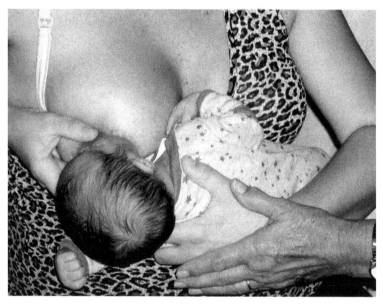

Transition hold – My hand positioned over Mum's hand demonstrates the ideal 'flat hand' rather than as shown, which is clutching baby. Mum is shaping her areola a little to assist baby to latch deeply. Notice her fingers are well away from the lower part of her breast where baby's chin needs to be firmly in contact as he latches.

Baby is positioned across Mother's body, with his hip positioned towards Mum's hip, rather than horizontally across her abdomen. Baby's whole body should be facing Mum's body. Baby is supported securely against her body with **her hand flat and firm across baby's shoulders** as she guides him upwards towards her breast. There should be no gap between her chest and baby's chest. As baby approaches the breast from underneath he will instinctively tilt his head back. This is the part which often worries parents, believing they must support baby's head. However, baby can be securely supported over the shoulders and body without holding his neck or the back of his head even with one finger. Having baby's head free to move is safe if he is well supported, and allows baby to follow his instincts to latch most effectively.

ATTACHING BABY TO BREASTFEED

WITH BABY POSITIONED as described above, Mother snuggles baby close so his lips and chin touch the breast below the areola (this results in baby's nose being opposite the top lip and nipple). It is the **chin being in firm contact** with the breast (not just nearby) that triggers baby's reflex to gape widely and "launch to latch". As baby's head tilts back and his chin contacts the breast the mother can support or shape her breast to help baby if needed. Mother is poised watching for baby to gape his mouth open wide. As baby gapes she hugs baby closer to her breast, enabling baby to take her areola and nipple deeply into his mouth. Baby pauses momentarily as the breast tissue and nipple are drawn into his mouth, and he begins sucking. When the mother feels he has established the latch she can gently take her hand away from the breast, and rest her arm under baby's back or shoulders.

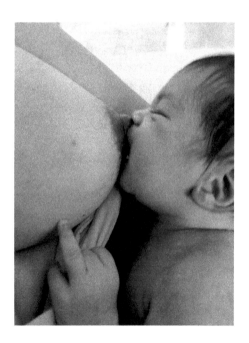

Baby is perfectly positioned with her **CHIN in contact** with the breast, and nipple opposite the top lip and nose. This **CONTACT** with the lower areola and breast stimulates baby's reflex to gape with a wide mouth.

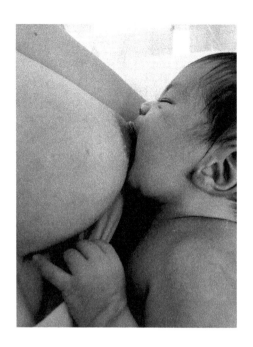

As Baby gapes widely she raises her top lip up and over the nipple; she simultaneously lowers her jaw with her tongue down as she draws the nipple and areola into her mouth, creating a vacuum inside her mouth.

When baby is latched her chin buries into the breast, her lips form a seal with her top lip in a neutral position (not curled out), and her nose is away from the breast so she can breathe easily. Baby's head is unrestricted. Mother's arm supports baby's shoulders securely as she snuggles her close to her body. Mother can rest back if she chooses so gravity helps baby stay comfortably latched.

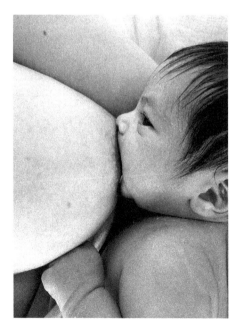

Having the baby's head tilted back enhances how widely baby can gape, enabling him to take in a maximum amount of breast tissue. This ensures optimal milk transfer and the most comfortable latch for baby and for mum. Some of the areola may be visible above baby's top lip, but most of the areola below the nipple will be inside baby's mouth.

The baby's head should never be held, even after latching successfully. Mothers sometimes do this to maintain the attachment, but it is unnecessary if baby is held firmly over the shoulders keeping the chin planted deeply into the breast, and with his body securely supported against mother's body. **Leaning back** during or after latching can be helpful as gravity helps keep baby in close contact with Mum. Babies resent having their head held as it is uncomfortable for them, and they resist head restriction by arching their body away from the breast during or shortly after attaching.

Most importantly the breastfeeding experience should be comfortable for both mother and baby. If the latch is painful for the Mother she must detach baby (by slipping her finger into the corner of his mouth to his gums to break the seal) and try again until she achieves a comfortable attachment. The nipple should look the same shape after the breastfeed as before it. If the nipple looks flattened, ridged or pointed ("lipstick shape") after the breastfeed the baby has not had enough breast tissue in his mouth. The nipple has been compressed against the roof of baby's mouth and the nipple will soon become sore and injured.

POSITIONS TO BREASTFEED BABY

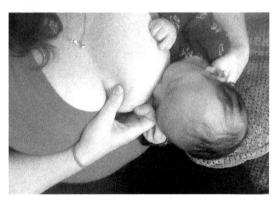

UNDERARM OR FOOTBALL HOLD: Baby is positioned beside Mum with her legs behind Mum's back. Baby is held over the shoulders only. Baby's body is turned to face Mum's hip. The deep latch allows her head to tilt back, with the nose clear. A pillow under Mum's arm/ elbow is helpful to support baby's weight.

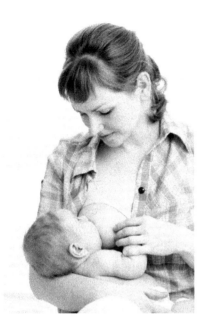

UPRIGHT: Baby is sitting in Mum's lap on an angle; baby's head is supported on Mum's arm and free to look upwards at Mum. This baby is in CRADLE HOLD

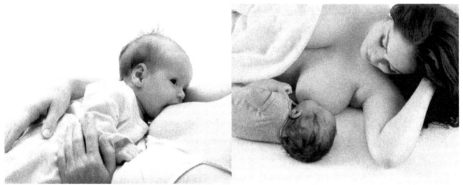

LAID BACK: Baby's body rests across Mum's body, and Baby's chin rests on the lower breast and her nose is clear. Baby's head is unrestricted.

SIDE-LYING: A good position to use when baby or Mum are sore and recovering from the birth, or Mum wants to rest while breastfeeding . Mother can also support baby with her hand over his shoulders to snuggle him close to her body.

HOW TO KNOW BABY IS FEEDING WELL

From feed to feed

During the breastfeed baby's whole jaw will move rhythmically with his suck/swallow/breath action. By listening for swallowing sounds, watching baby's feeding action and even counting how many sucks baby does before swallowing, Mothers can gauge how well baby is drinking. Baby needs to maintain the head comfortably tilted back position throughout the breastfeed, which enables him to swallow the milk comfortably and efficiently – just the same as adults need to tilt their heads back to drink from a bottle.

Baby's cheeks should appear full and his lower lip will be flanged downwards, while the upper lip will rest in a neutral or slightly everted position. The top lip does not need to be flanged outwards. If baby's cheeks are dimpling inwards as he sucks he does not have his tongue positioned correctly, and he is not really feeding effectively.

The Mother should take notice of the rhythm and depth of his jaw movement and the pauses between suck/swallow bursts. It is a normal pattern of feeding for baby to suck/swallow, then pause, and as baby gets fuller the sucks get shorter and the pauses get longer. As baby nears the end of that phase of the feed he may rest as he pauses, his chin may tremble or mum may feel little fluttery sucks. Baby may partially or fully release his latch, and appear satisfied and probably sleepy. **How well** the baby fed is more important than **how long** baby was at the breast. A baby can take a large volume of milk in a short time (5 or 10 minutes) if he is optimally positioned and attached, whereas a poorly positioned and attached baby may drink far less milk even when he has been at the breast for 30 minutes or more.

Mother can also be guided by how her breast feels after the feed to indicate how much milk baby drank. Does the breast feel softer or less heavy than it did at the beginning of the feed? As already explained, each breastfeed is usually comprised of a few phases or instalments. Young babies particularly need to take each 'meal' in a few stages, with rest times in between each stage to allow comfortable digestion. If possible, return baby to the starting breast at least once before offering the second breast. Baby will show you he is full by appearing comfortable and satisfied, and probably look 'milk drunk' and sleepy. If he settles easily after burping and nappy changes if needed, he has had enough. If he doesn't, he probably needs a bit more breastfeeding – sometimes it is only a few extra minutes of suckling which satisfies baby. Trust your baby's cues, and you will soon gain confidence about judging when he has completed his breastfeed.

From day to day
Baby's output – his wees and poos – are a reliable guide to whether he is taking sufficient volumes of breastmilk at each feed. In the first day of baby's life we expect one wee and a few black 'meconium' poos; on his second day we expect two wees and a few poos which may become brownish 'transitional'. From day 3 we expect three wees and the poos to be changing to yellow-ish 'mature' poos. When baby is 4-5 days old and mother's milk has 'come in' his output becomes established at around 8 nappies per 24 hours. If baby is feeding well many of his nappies will be wet and pooey, and they may total more than 8 per day. The breastfed baby's mustard-yellow coloured poo is quite runny or like fluffy mousse and it may have little grainy looking bits in it – this is all normal. When a baby is taking adequate amounts of breastmilk he will produce at least **3 poos every 24 hours.** His wees will look pale yellow coloured, and some nappies should be quite heavily wet.

If a baby is not taking adequate breastmilk volumes the amount of poo reduces, however the wet nappies continue. If a breastfed baby less than 6 weeks old produces less than two poos each 24 hours this is an early indication that the baby may not be obtaining enough breastmilk. This situation needs to be checked by a midwife, child health nurse or doctor as soon as it is recognised. If baby's output fits the normal description above you can be assured baby is getting enough breastmilk.

After about 6 weeks of age baby's anal sphincter begins to work more effectively and can hold on to poo for longer, so it is normal for these older babies to poo less frequently. As long as the urine output continues to require 6 or more nappies per day, baby feeds regularly (6-8 or more times each 24 hours) settles well between feeds and his weight gain is consistently good (150gms or more per week), the reduced poo output is not a concern. I emphasise, less than 2 poos per day is NOT normal for a baby less than 6 weeks old.

From week to week
Newborn babies should be weighed weekly for the first month or two of their lives. A well fed baby will regain his birthweight within the first two weeks of life, and continue to grow in length, head circumference and weight over the following months. Baby will have his most rapid period of growth during the first three months gaining 150-200 grams per week, however weight gains will vary from week to week and also from baby to baby. Mother's milk production peaks during this time at about 750-800 mls per day, and the constituents of her breastmilk are continually adjusting automatically to her baby's changing requirements as he grows. The rate of baby's weight gain slows down by about 50% after about three months but a well baby's physical growth and development continues to astonish and reassure his parents that they are doing a great job in their new roles.

Breastmilk provides the very best nutrition for your baby. Baby will benefit most if he is exclusively breastfed for the first six months of his life (ie no other foods or milk except breastmilk). A breastfed baby does not need additional water because breastmilk contains all the fluid baby needs for hydration. Extra water given orally does not provide any nutrition, and it makes baby less hungry and can cause baby to miss out on feeding which he actually needs. A breastfed baby is likely to feed more often during warm weather to quench his thirst, just as adults drink more frequently in warm weather for the same reason.

Extra water can be given when baby starts solid foods which the World Health Organisation recommends can be offered around 6 months of age. "Baby Led Weaning" is an excellent way to introduce family foods. Ideally breastmilk continues to be the main source of nutrition for baby during the second half of his first year of life, and beyond as it continues to provide valuable immune factors throughout toddlerhood. Milk remains the main form of nutrition for babies up to 12 months of age, even if they are eating some family foods.

Mother's Diet

Advice about a breastfeeding mother's diet abounds with myths, and breastfeeding mothers often believe they must deprive themselves of certain foods and drinks to avoid problems. Here is the good news – a breastfeeding mother's diet should include all the usual healthy food components such as fruit and vegetables, grains, meat and fish, and dairy foods that she usually enjoys, and plenty of water. Both Mother and baby require nutrition around the clock, and the lactating mother requires more caloric intake than at any other time In her life. A regular diet of healthy foods and plenty of water is essential for the wellbeing of a breastfeeding Mother and her baby.

The common-sense recommendation of 'everything in moderation' applies here, so excessive amounts of any food or drink should be avoided. Yes, Mum can have a cup of coffee, a spicy curry, and even a small serve of chocolate if that is her desire – but not three cups of coffee and a whole block of chocolate! If a breastfeeding Mum would like a glass of wine or other alcoholic drink she should breastfeed her baby first, **then** have a drink. The amount of alcohol which is in the mother's breastmilk is equivalent to her blood alcohol level, and the elimination of the alcohol from her system will be the same for her breastmilk as for her bloodstream. If a Mum follows this advice her body will eliminate the alcohol from her system over several hours, and by the time baby needs to be breastfed again she can do so knowing she is doing him no harm. (Remember, everything in moderation!)

Dairy foods eaten in moderation are fine, but if baby develops signs of digestive and skin problems cow's milk proteins in breastmilk are likely to be suspected. Elimination of dairy from Mother's diet may be recommended by her doctor or lactation consultant. A 2 week period of eliminating dairy from mother's diet is usually long enough to determine if the baby's discomfort WAS due to dairy/Cow's Milk Protein (CMP), or not.

The most common foods which might cause discomfort for baby via mother's milk are cruciferous vegetables (cabbage, cauliflower, brussel sprouts, broccoli, peas), so eating only small servings of these vegetables is probably a good idea until the Mother knows her baby copes with these foods in her diet. Everything in moderation.

There are some foods which are known to support and enhance breastmilk production (called lactogenic foods). These include rolled oats (as porridge or as an ingredient in cookies), a coffee substitute drink called Caro which is derived from barley, and foods containing Omega 3 fatty acids. Brewer's Yeast and some herbs are also believed to enhance breastmilk production (eg Fenugreek, Blessed Thistle) and are found in a multitude of combinations sold as breastfeeding support products. Women who are asthmatic or diabetic, or allergic to peanuts or chick peas should be very cautious and seek medical advice before taking herbal breastfeeding products.

ALTERNATE METHODS OF FEEDING BABY

Finger feeding

If baby has problems latching to breastfeed in the early hours and days of life, colostrum, breastmilk or formula may be offered by finger feeds. To feed baby this way a clean finger – usually the index finger or the thumb is gently introduced to baby's mouth with the finger nail resting on the baby's tongue and the fleshy part of the finger facing upwards toward the roof of baby's mouth. Gentle pressure and stroking will stimulate baby to close his lips around the finger and start to suck, with the tongue extended forward "cupping" the finger and forming a vacuum. When baby is sucking some colostrum or milk is given by syringe beside the finger, which baby swallows down. This is an easy and effective means of getting nutrition into the baby temporarily until the baby's feeding skills improve. A Lactation Consultant or Midwife should always be involved in assisting the mother and baby to establish normal feeding as soon as possible.

Cup feeding

Babies can be fed from a small cup if necessary as a temporary alternative to breast or bottle feeding. Surprisingly, even premature babies can do this if offered correctly. The baby needs to be alert and interested in feeding. Baby should be wrapped in a bunny rug or thin towel so their hands are kept out of the way, and a bib or small towel placed in front as there will be some dribbling.

A small clean cup like a medicine cup or egg cup can be used, half filled with milk. With baby sat upright and well supported the cup is placed at baby's lower lip, and tilted so milk just touches the lips. Baby will extend her tongue forward as for finger feeding and lap at the milk. The cup should be kept in place at the lips while baby laps and pauses, then laps again, tipping gently to keep the milk accessible by baby's tongue action. Do not pour milk into baby's mouth as she may inhale some milk and aspirate it into her lungs. This video by Global Health Media demonstrates how to feed a small baby by cup: **https://globalhealthmedia.org/videos/cup-feeding-your-small-baby/**

Spoon feeding a newborn and hand expression of breastmilk are demonstrated in this **video: Hand expression of breastmilk - https://med.stanford.edu/ newborns/professional-education/breastfeeding/hand-expressing-milk.html**

Bottle feeding
It is a fact of our modern lives that most babies will be fed by a bottle and teat at some time. Breastfeeding mothers may decide to give some breastmilk by bottle once their supply is well established for a variety of reasons. They may be planning a night away from baby, or returning to work and needing to be able to leave the baby in someone else's care for a period of time. It can be difficult to get a fully breastfed baby to accept a bottle and teat if it is not introduced by 3 or 4 months of age, so offering baby an occasional bottle feed after about 6 weeks of age can help baby adapt to this alternative feeding method more easily.   It is important to understand that giving a breastfed baby frequent feeds by bottle and teat can 'derail' the baby from breastfeeding. Babies who are "mixed fed" breast and bottle can begin to prefer bottle feeds as it is easier (called "flow preference"), because it requires less physical effort to bottle feed than to breastfeed.

PACED BOTTLE FEEDING AKA RESPONSIVE BOTTLE FEEDING

"RESPONSIVE BOTTLE FEEDING is defined as "encouraging mothers to tune in to feeding cues and to hold their babies close during feeds. Offering the bottle in response to feeding cues, gently inviting the baby to take the teat, pacing the feeds and avoiding forcing the baby to finish the feed can all help to make the experience as acceptable and stress-free for the baby as possible, as well as reducing the risk of overfeeding. Other tips for responsive bottle feeding include keeping the bottle horizontal during the feeding to minimize gulping and overfeeding and allowing for frequent pauses that occur naturally during breastfeeding. Responsive feeding allows the baby to be "in control" of the feeding and is related to better self-regulation of food impacting the later possibility of obesity." **Source: https://icea.org/responsive-feeding/**

The traditional image we have of bottle feeding a baby typically has baby laid back resting in the crook of the carer's arm, with the bottle and teat held at an upright angle, which fills the teat with milk. It was believed this positioning ensured baby did not take in air while suckling the bottle teat. When bottle feeds are delivered this way the milk is usually ingested quickly, and the baby has no control over the rate she takes the milk, or the volume swallowed. We now know this traditional bottle feeding method can lead to overfilling baby which can increase posseting and vomiting, and baby becomes accustomed to the sensation of a very full stomach. Research indicates this lack of control affects baby's ability to recognise comfortable fullness and self-regulate by ceasing or pausing a feed, in the way a baby self-regulates intake when breastfeeding. Instead, baby is usually coaxed to finish all the milk offered in the bottle, which can lead to overfeeding.

The paced bottle feeding technique is almost the opposite of the traditional method described above. Instead, baby is held in a more upright position, and the bottle is held in a position horizontal to the floor with the teat half-filled with milk. The baby's cues, and suck/swallow/pause pattern are observed closely. The bottle is tilted back slightly each time baby pauses, allowing a brief period without milk flow, until baby reinitiates the suckling action and milk is offered again. Regardless of what type of teat is used, pacing the intake of milk to correspond with baby's sucking and pause pattern mimics the natural sequences observed in breastfeeding babies. The baby is then able to take the milk at a rate that is comfortable for him, and can respond to his feelings of fullness by pausing or ceasing the feeding. A paced bottle feed is likely to be given in a few instalments in response to baby's cues, similar to how a baby takes a breastfeed. Allowing for burps, cuddles, nappy changes and rests the time taken to complete a feed will be similar to a breastfeed – about an hour. Most importantly, the baby will be in control of the volume ingested, and can develop his self-regulation responses. The baby is also more likely to digest the feed more comfortably too.

This YouTube video demonstrates paced bottle feeding: "The Milk Mob – Paced Bottle Feeding" **https://youtu.be/OGPm5SpLxXY**

BOTTLES AND TEATS

THERE ARE NUMEROUS BOTTLES and teats on the market which claim to provide a delivery system which is like breastfeeding, however in my experience most do not even come close. To maintain breastfeeding it is very important for baby to be offered a teat which closely simulates the way breast milk flows from the breast in response to baby's tongue and jaw action, which initiates and controls the flow of milk. The only teat I have found which simulates baby's natural suckling and swallowing action is the *Pigeon Peristaltic Plus Wide-Neck* "Y"cut teat, **when the feed is given using the "Paced Bottle Feeding Technique".**

For parents wanting to introduce occasional bottle feeds to a breastfed baby I suggest you buy one small Pigeon Peristaltic Plus Wide-Neck Bottle which comes with a standard teat (with holes) S or SS (slow flow) and one packet of **Pigeon Peristaltic Plus Wide-Neck "Y" teats Size "M" (3).** The label states these teats are designed for babies over 3 months old, but I have found them to be fine for well younger babies who have a normal ability to suck.   Pigeon bottles come in both standard neck and wide-neck options – it is the wide-neck which I prefer because the wider shape of the teat comfortably allows baby to maintain a wide gape while feeding. The Pigeon "Y" cut teat only allows milk to flow when the baby uses his jaw and tongue in a similar way to when he breastfeeds. Each time baby pauses, the little Y cut closes; when sucking is reinitiated the Y-cut allows milk to flow again. There is a small vent in the teat which should be positioned under baby's nose to ensure correct orientation of the Y cut outlet. Pigeon bottles and teats are suitable to use for breastmilk or formula feeding. In my experience most other wide-based bottles are too wide, and baby's mouth tends to slip back to the tip of the teat, causing pursed lips and minimal jaw activity – like sucking a straw. The Lansinoh brand wide neck teat is very similar in shape to the Pigeon Soft Touch wide neck teat.

CLEANING AND STERILISING BOTTLES AND TEATS AND EXPRESSING EQUIPMENT PARTS

RINSE BOTTLES AND TEATS with COLD water immediately after use. All bottles teats and parts should then be thoroughly washed in warm soapy water using a bottle brush to clean the insides, and rinsed with hot water. Advice about sterilising bottles has changed over recent years. Some health authorities now advise sterilising of bottles and teats is unnecessary if they are thoroughly cleaned as above, and not used by more than one baby.

For parents who choose to sterilise their baby's equipment, boiling or steaming is still the most effective method. For occasional use boiling a bottle, teat and caps for two minutes in a saucepan and allowing it to cool before removing the items (with clean hands) is the simplest option. Allow the parts to drain and air dry on a clean tea towel or sheet of paper towel, then assemble and store in in your fridge ready for use.   Microwave steriliser containers are cheap to buy and quick to use, providing a handy alternative if you have several bottles and parts to sterilise. Electric sterilisers are effective but more expensive and take up more space in your kitchen.   Chemical sterilising methods are no longer recommended.

Formula Feeding

In years past it was common practise for a number of bottles to be made up at once, so they were ready to use when needed. The current advice is to make up each bottle of formula just before baby needs to be fed. This recommendation is due to the increased risk of bacterial growth in the formula after boiled water is added and it is stored, even if the bottles are refrigerated. Powdered Infant Formula (PIF) is not a sterile product, and any powdered milk can contain contaminants such as Cronobacter Sakazakii and Salmonella. For this reason **the World Health Organisation (WHO)** recommends using hot water no less than 70 degrees Celsius to make up powdered infant formula as these bacteria will be killed by the hot water if they are present in the powder. (Boiling water in a jug and waiting 20 minutes will reduce the water temperature to 70 degrees Celsius). Some Australian health authorities have not yet adopted this recommendation and still advise making formula up with cooled boiled water. Parents can decide for themselves which advice to follow.

If hot water is used the bottle of formula needs to be cooled under a running tap or sat in cold water to cool it to lukewarm temperature before giving. Formula made with cooled boiled water may be warmed by sitting in a mug or jug of warm water. Always check the temperature of the bottle of formula by shaking it, then dripping some milk onto the inside of your wrist to check it is not too hot for baby. Heating baby's bottle in a microwave oven is not recommended because the heat can be unevenly dispersed with some parts of the milk overheated, and there are also concerns about microwaves causing changes to the nutrients in the formula.

Good hygiene is essential when handling any of baby's feeding equipment. Hands must be washed and counter surfaces should be wiped clean before beginning to make up each bottle of formula. It is also not advisable to keep the powder scoop in the tin after use, as it is handled many times during the life of the tin of powdered formula which increases the risk of germs being transferred to the powder.

Appliances are now available which make up formula bottles automatically (almost). If you choose to use one of these ensure sufficiently hot water is dispensed to meet the WHO recommendations. All compartments where powdered formula is held must be kept very clean, as pathogens could be harboured inside the various parts which come in contact with the milk. Also follow the recommended proportions of formula to water carefully.

Wide-neck bottles are easier to use to make up formula feeds than the narrow neck bottles, and easier to clean. Plastic bottles for babies are now BPA free (not made from plastics which could leach toxins into the milk when heated) and are practical for daily use, however some parents may prefer glass bottles. If a milky film collects inside teats, rubbing the inside with a pinch of kitchen salt prior to washing will cleanse the teat thoroughly. Which teats will suit your baby is really a matter of experimentation. Small babies tend to manage slow-flow teats better than fast flow teats, however medium flow teats may be better for premature babies or those with a weak suck. The paced bottle feeding technique is recommended for babies of all ages.

Choosing Formula

Most infant formula is cows' milk based with various additives. Formulas vary for babies of different ages from Birth onwards. First infant milk is whey dominant, which means it is designed to be easily digested by a normal healthy newborn baby. Formula which is designed for older or hungrier babies are usually casein dominant, which is harder to digest than whey. Goats' Milk infant formula has also been developed and available for sale on supermarket shelves. Manufacturers of both cows' and goats' milk infant formula in Australia and New Zealand must comply with the Code (updated in 2021) which details composition and safety standards to ensure that the nutritional requirements of infants are met. **https://www.foodstandards.gov. au/Infant formula**

The directions on the tin are a guide of how many scoops to add to the recommended volume of water to provide the correct strength of formula for the baby of a certain age. It is important to follow these directions exactly. The amount of milk taken by a baby may vary from feed to feed, and any leftover milk should always be thrown away when baby has finished the feed.

If you need to make a bottle of formula for baby when you are not at home, you should take the sterilised bottle with the measured amount of boiled water, and the powder in a separate container. Handy flip-top holders are available to carry measured portions of powdered infant formula, which can be added to the water and mixed just before use. Make sure the formula carriers are emptied and washed regularly too!

The amount of milk to offer babies at different ages can be varied before the baby reaches the next age level on the can's directions, if the baby seems to need more. I have met parents who thought they could not feed their two week old baby the amount suggested for 3-4 weeks of age, even though the baby was clearly still hungry and her weight gain was not great. Be discerning, and be flexible. Be guided by your baby's feeding cues and signs of being satisfied, rather than only offering the suggested amounts written on the tin. Consult with your Child Health Nurse if you are uncertain about what volumes of formula your baby needs.

Specialised formula milks such as those for low birthweight or preterm babies should be used strictly in consultation with a paediatrician. Babies with problems such as allergies or reflux should also have their feeding guided by a doctor or paediatrician to ensure a proper diagnosis is made and appropriate treatments are prescribed in addition to specialised infant formula. This also applies to the use of rice and soya based infant formulas.

Giving bottle feeds
It is important how a baby is held during bottle feeding. Breast fed babies spend lots of time in close contact with their mothers, allowing time for them to gaze at one another, enhancing bonding. Bottle fed babies can miss out on this physical and eye contact time, particularly as bottle feed can be completed in a shorter time than a full breast feed. (See Paced Bottle Feeding). Alternating which side baby is held while bottle feeding simulates the natural variation of positioning which occurs when mothers switch sides while breastfeeding.

Start the bottle feed by stroking the baby's lips with the teat to coax her to open her mouth. Put the teat into baby's mouth resting gently on her tongue, allowing her to gape and flange her lips around the wider part of the teat. Refer to the information about Paced Bottle Feeding for guidance about feeding technique. Watch baby's response to the milk going into her throat and how comfortably she swallows. The flow should be steady but not fast, allowing baby to suck, swallow and breathe without struggling with any part of the process. Expect baby to take rest periods, or even a nap, between the instalments of the bottle feed. Swap sides during the feed, similar to how baby alternates sides during breastfeeding. Bottles should **never** be propped for a baby of any age to drink unattended.

Water – Breastfed babies **do not** require extra water even in hot weather. Breastmilk contains exactly the right amount of water to meet baby's hydration needs, however baby may feed more frequently in hot weather to quench his thirst. Giving water to a breastfed baby makes baby's stomach feel full and may cause him to refuse a breastfeed, missing out on the nutrients he needs.

Babies under 6 months of age are not able to safely process water alone due to the immaturity of their kidneys. Giving water can lead to a serious condition called water intoxication, which can be fatal. Formula fed babies may need extra water as a supplement to formula feeds in hot weather. This may be given as separate sips of boiled water. Extra water should not added in a bottle of formula because it will alter the concentration of the formula and baby would receive less nutrients.

Burping

Burping is not compulsory! Burping babies is a Western society obsession, not seen in most other cultures. If baby does not easily volunteer a burp or two, don't worry – the wind will come out one way or another. Parents may think the baby MUST burp before resuming the feed and can spend much time trying to get it to happen. If it is not worrying the baby, it doesn't need to worry the parents if the baby doesn't burp on cue. Some babies burp easily and a lot, others hardly ever – this is normal. Responding to baby's cues to continue the feed is more important than getting a burp up.

Many babies will have a burp to bring up during or after a full breastfeed or bottle feed. Baby may begin to wriggle or squirm around during the feed when they have some wind making them uncomfortable. A burp can be helped along by sitting baby <u>upright with a straight back</u>, and can be **gently** rubbed or patted on the back while waiting for the wind to come up. Alternatively baby can be placed upright over a parent's RIGHT shoulder, with the baby's tummy held comfortably against the parent's body. Gentle rubbing or patting will usually result in a burp coming up, if it needs to. Avoid thumping or banging baby's back to help with burping, as this is likely to increase spitting up, posseting or vomiting. Watch the **NewBaby101 video: "<u>How to breastfeed Baby</u>"** to see another gentle method of helping baby to burp.

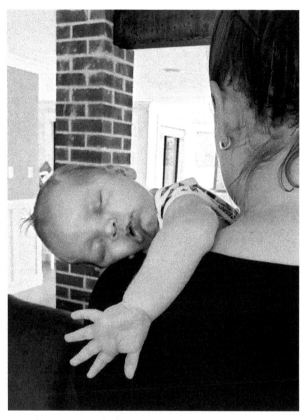

When baby is full and satisfied he often signals this with relaxed arms and "fanned" fingers.

TOPIC 5
FEEDTIME (Part 2)
Concerns and Problems

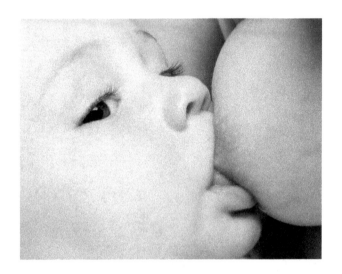

NEWBORN BABIES WHO DON'T FEED WELL

WELL NEWBORN BABIES ARE naturally inclined to breastfeed shortly after birth.
They usually have a long sleep after the birth and taking their first breastfeed
– this is normal. They then wake up and feed every few hours, seeking and
obtaining the rich protective colostrum nature provides for their survival, and
activation of their gastrointestinal system and pristine gut microbiome.

Pain relief given to the Mother during labour such as narcotic medications
(Pethidine, Morphine) and epidural drugs given over an extended period
will pass across the placenta to the baby and can significantly affect baby's
responses after birth. Babies who are exposed to these drugs during labour
may take several days to completely eliminate them from their bodies, and
consequently are often sleepy and slow to respond normally by feeding
frequently in the early days of life. Babies may also have swallowed fluids

during the birth process, and may have mucousy vomits in the early days of life which also makes them less inclined to feed well. Babies born by caesarean section are often more mucousy because their chest and lungs have not been stimulated by the natural squeezing process of vaginal birth.

Babies who are not interested in feeding need to be given frequent small amounts of colostrum which can be hand expressed by the Mother and given to baby by syringe or spoon. Doing so will reduce the likelihood of baby becoming dehydrated or losing excessive weight during the first 3 days of life. All babies lose some weight after birth, but then begin to gain weight as feeding progresses. If a baby loses more than 10% of his birthweight in the first 3 days of life his electrolyte balance may be affected which can seriously harm the baby.

Birth trauma caused by an assisted birth (vacuum extraction or forceps) can make baby very sore and uncomfortable during breastfeeding. Mothers should try various breastfeeding positions to find how baby is most comfortable to enable baby to breastfeed effectively. The side-lying position often works best for these Mothers and babies. Mothers should ask for assistance from Midwives while in hospital to ensure baby is feeding frequently, effectively and comfortably. A home visit from a Lactation Consultant can also be very helpful for mothers whose babies are still recovering from the effects of their birth and needing assistance with breastfeeds.

Problems latching
Every mother and baby are a unique pair. Babies may encounter problems attaching to the breast if the mother has flat or inverted nipples, or large heavy breasts, or if baby is compromised by pain or a physical problem which makes feeding difficult or tiring. Many factors can be associated with latching problems and expert breastfeeding assessment and advice is essential for each individual case.

A Nipple Shield can be a helpful temporary tool for a mother and baby struggling to latch to breastfeed. These are designed particularly for women with flat or inverted nipples, and may enable their babies to latch for breastfeeds which often draws the nipple out somewhat, and over time baby may then manage to latch without the nipple shield. Likewise, mothers whose babies have had setbacks after birth and breastfeeding has been delayed, can be helped to establish breastfeeding with the use of a nipple shield. It is important the correct size nipple shield is used, which matches the size of the mother's nipple, not the size of the baby's mouth. It is a common mistake to use a small nipple shield (16mm) because baby is new and small, when the mother's nipple size suits a medium (20mm) or large (24mm) shield. This often results in discomfort and injury to the mother's nipple, and can impair effective milk transfer.

As mentioned, a nipple shield can be a helpful TEMPORARY tool. Babies can become dependent on the shield over time and it may be difficult to stop using them for breastfeeds. One way to wean from nipple shield use can be to start a breastfeed with the shield in place, and when baby suckles well and the milk starts flowing, remove the shield and try re-latching baby without the shield. If it doesn't work, return the nipple shield and try it again at another feed. Aim to gradually do more parts of each feed without the shield, rather than changing things all at once.

How the shield is applied is also important. There are various brands of nipple shields, and application technique can differ according to their design. The New Baby 101 video (below) demonstrates how to apply a Medela Nipple Shield. I recommend positioning the flanged side of the Medela shield opposite baby's nose and the cutaway section under the nipple. This allows baby's mouth and tongue to touch the areola and also draw in some tissue. When the shield is positioned with the cutaway opposite the nose (as described in the instructions) the flange of the shield creates a barrier between baby's mouth and the breast tissue, which can impair and reduce breast stimulation and milk transfer. **https://youtu.be/u7EHuQ4HOxQ**

TONGUE TIE (ANKYLOGLOSSIA)

A FRENULUM UNDER THE TONGUE it is a remnant of oral anatomy creation during the embryological stage of baby's development. As an embryo the tongue is fused to the floor of the mouth. It separates by a process called apoptosis (cell death) which is programmed to happen as the tongue develops. Sometimes this natural separation process is incomplete, resulting in a remnant membrane. If the remnant tissue (frenulum) is short, thick or attached close to the tip of the tongue in may limit tongue movement and affect tongue function.

About 5-8% of babies have a condition called tongue-tie which may contribute to problems attaching or sustaining the latch to feed. In babies with tongue-tie the membrane of tissue under the tongue (called the frenulum) attaches to the underside of the tongue and secures in the floor of the mouth or lower gum line. The frenulum can limit tongue movement, particularly lift and extension of the tongue making latching difficult and feeding very tiring. However seeing a frenulum under the tongue does not necessarily mean baby will have breastfeeding problems.

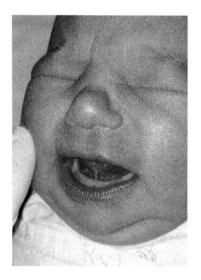

Tongue-ties need to be individually assessed by an expert such as a Lactation Consultant or Midwife, who after observing a breast feed and examining the baby's mouth may recommend a procedure called **frenotomy**. This is a very simple procedure which is usually performed by a Paediatrician or credentialed Lactation Consultant using sterile scissors. It involves snipping the thin piece of tissue (frenulum) to release the tongue so it can function normally. No anaesthetic is needed, in most cases there is little or no bleeding and the breastfeeding feeding problem is resolved immediately. Laser division of tongue-ties is not superior to using scissors. It is expensive and invasive, much slower and more likely to cause formation of scar tissue. The Academy of Breastfeeding Medicine and the Australian Dental Association advise against division of the infant frenulum by laser. **https://pubmed.ncbi.nlm.nih.gov/33852342/**

Upper Lip Ties
In the majority of babies (93.3%) the upper lip frenulum (called the maxillary or labial frenulum) is seen under the upper lip joining on to the upper gum. It is a feature of normal oral anatomy. Some practitioners, particularly some dentists, may recommend cutting an upper lip frenulum often using a laser instrument, to assist breastfeeding. There is absolutely no scientific evidence to support this procedure. The upper lip only needs to rest in a neutral position or slightly curved outwards to seal the breast in the baby's mouth, and to function in unison with the tongue and lower jaw during breastfeeding.

The appearance of the upper lip frenulum changes over time with growth and development. The frenulum gets smaller, thinner, and will insert higher up on the gum line as the first teeth erupt. By the time a child has permanent teeth the upper lip frenulum looks very different to how it looked as an infant. If a gap is present between the top teeth (dyastema), this is often an inherited feature of another family members' teeth. The Australian Dental Association advise the upper lip frenulum should only be divided if problems arise with food becoming trapped there, and only after mature dentition is complete after 12 years of age.

Parents may also be concerned about Buccal or Cheek ties which they have heard may contribute to "oral restrictions". There is no evidence to indicate these frenula require division if they are observed. Labial and Buccal frenula form the "scaffolding" of baby's oral anatomy and are there for that structural purpose. For more information about the treatment and potential over-treatment of tongue and lip ties watch this video from the Australian Breastfeeding Association. **https://vimeo.com/442896299 https://www.breastfeeding.asn.au/bf-info/to**

Jaundice
Most newborn babies have some jaundice (yellow-ish skin) temporarily, from Day 2 to Day 7 of life. This is called physiological jaundice and happens as a

result of baby's natural adjustment to life outside the womb. The unborn baby needs more red blood cells to carry oxygen than he needs after birth when he is taking oxygen into his system through his lungs. As excess red blood cells are broken down by the body and one of the molecules which break off is a fat soluble yellow-pigment molecule called **bilirubin**. The baby's liver and kidneys can't process all of the bilirubin at once and some molecules find their way to the fatty tissue under the skin (making the skin look yellow) and also the fatty tissue of the brain making the baby sleepy.

If the condition is mild and baby continues to wake up for feeds every few hours, and does plenty of wee and poo to excrete the bilirubin molecules, jaundice does not cause any problems. If the baby becomes very sleepy as a result of excess circulating bilirubin he should be woken for feeds if he does not self-waken, and he may need stimulation and prompting to continue feeding properly after latching. Positioning baby in an area of the home where white light comes in, and exposing baby's head and upper body to the light during the day will also help her body to eliminate the excessive bilirubin from her system. Note: baby should not be exposed to direct sunlight!

New parents need to be aware of the importance of baby taking frequent and effective feeds if he is jaundiced. If baby is allowed to sleep for long periods the bilirubin builds up in the bloodstream, skin and brain cells, and is not readily eliminated from baby's system via baby's output (wee and poo), which slow down with infrequent feeding. If baby is too sleepy to breastfeed he must be offered milk by finger feeds or bottle and medical help sought immediately. Blood tests may need to be done to determine if the bilirubin levels in baby's system are excessive, and if they are high phototherapy (light) treatment must be commenced without delay, as jaundice in its advanced form can be life-threatening to baby if untreated.

HICCUPS

SOME BABIES GET HICCUPS OFTEN – others do not. Both are normal. When parents inquire about a newborn's hiccups I ask "Did the baby have hiccups a lot when he was inside you?" Most often the answer is "Yes" – and my response is "Well he will be a hiccup-y baby on the outside too". Hiccups are just a reaction of the baby's immature diaphragm responding to the fullness of the stomach after a feed. When in the womb the baby swallows amniotic fluid, filling the stomach which stimulates the diaphragm in the same way. Hiccups concern parents much more than they concern the baby. Laying baby on her tummy for a few minutes or giving a bit more milk will usually settle hiccups.

SNEEZING

Newborn babies often sneeze and parents may worry unnecessarily that baby has a cold. Babies' noses are often squashed and squeezed during the birth process, and may have one or both nostrils partly blocked until the nasal tissue moves and adjusts to life outside the womb. During feeding some milk may sit in the back of the throat and nasal passages and it is a natural reflex for baby to sneeze in response to this temporary irritation. In most cases sneezing is a natural occurrence for babies just as it is with adults.

The exception to this is if baby has been exposed to a person (usually another child) who has a cold or respiratory illness, and baby is showing signs of being unwell such as poor feeding, unsettled behaviour, elevated temperature, or sleeping for excessive times. The most common germ which causes young children's infections is **Respiratory Syncytial Virus** or **RSV** which will cause cold-type symptoms in the older child, but can be life threatening in a young baby. If a young baby is displaying the symptoms above she should be checked by a doctor as soon as possible.

BLISTER ON BABY'S TOP LIP

BABY MAY DEVELOP A 'sucking blister' on their top lip, especially in the early days of frequent breastfeeding. This may indicate baby has not been attached to the breast in the most effective way which has resulted in some friction as baby's upper lip slides on the breast during suckling. Improvement of the positioning and attachment technique will result in a more effective latch, reducing the movement and friction as baby feeds. Nevertheless, many young babies develop a "sucking blister" on their top lip without any apparent feeding problems, in which case it is nothing to worry about and will disappear on its own.

CONSTIPATION

A FULLY BREASTFED BABY cannot become constipated. The breastfed baby's poo is always soft or runny, and the chemistry of the breastfed baby's gut cannot create a firm stool (poo).

A baby being fed with formula can become constipated very easily, and this is the most common reason parents change baby to a different formula. One traditional remedy for constipation in a formula fed baby is to mix about 20mls of warm boiled water with one teaspoon of brown sugar, and give this to baby by bottle. One dose should be sufficient to enable baby to pass a bowel motion in a day or so. Parents should seek advice from their Child Health Nurse or Doctor if their baby has problems with constipation rather than trying to sort the problem out by trying various brands of formula or over the counter medications.

If a young breastfed baby (less than a month old) is pooing infrequently, or misses a day or more it indicates baby may not be transferring sufficient breastmilk. Baby's weight gains should be closely monitored, and help with breastfeeding technique and assessment by a lactation consultant or child health nurse is recommended. The use of suppositories to stimulate bowel activity is not advised.

Anal Stenosis – a small number of babies show signs of discomfort during bowel actions and visibly strain and may become distressed while doing poo, even though the poo is soft when baby finally manages to empty his bowel. This could be because of a tight anal sphincter muscle called anal stenosis, which makes passing bowel motions hard work for the baby and a distressing time for the parents too. Treatment is quite simple and involves a procedure of gently dilating the anal sphincter muscle, which is done by a GP or paediatrician.

ORAL THRUSH

ORAL THRUSH CAN OCCUR in breastfed and bottle fed babies. Patches of white plaque will be seen on baby's tongue, inside the cheeks or roof of the mouth. Baby may be irritable and uncomfortable during feeds if they have oral thrush, and this fungal infection is readily transferred to the mother's areola and nipples. This will appear as a red irritation which may also be shiny on the nipple and areola, or just general tenderness without any obvious skin changes. Baby may also develop a red skin irritation on his bottom. Mother or baby can be vulnerable to developing thrush after having a course of antibiotics.

Both baby and mother need to be treated if thrush symptoms appear on either or both mother and baby. Scrupulous hand hygiene should be observed and feeding equipment, dummies and anything else which comes in contact with baby's mouth must be thoroughly cleaned and sterilised. Mother's bras, towels and non-disposable breast pads should be washed in warm water and dried in the sunshine.

Medications to treat symptoms of thrush are available 'over the counter' at pharmacies. Miconazole gel (Daktarin) can be applied to baby's mouth, and Clotrimazole or Miconazole cream can be applied to mother's breast and baby's bottom. Some pharmacists may decline selling Daktarin to parents of young babies, and may want written confirmation from a GP before dispensing it. Follow the directions and continue treatment for at least 7 days. Seek advice from a Lactation Consultant, Child Health Nurse or Doctor if thrush symptoms persist or reoccur.

VOMITING AND POSSETING

BABIES WILL OFTEN bring up a little of the milk (called posseting) when they bring up a burp. It is a common and benign (nothing to worry about) condition, caused by the immature sphincter muscle at the top of baby's stomach which does not close very firmly, and when some wind comes up a little milk comes too. Provided a newborn baby is gaining weight and does normal amounts of wee and poo (a minimum of 2 poo nappies each 24 hours, and 5 wet nappies) bringing up some milk is not a problem except for the extra washing it may create. Babies who vomit often but are unperturbed by it are called "happy chuckers". It is NEVER normal for a baby to vomit bile (dark green coloured vomit). If this happens baby should be seen by a doctor as soon as possible.

Some babies are inclined to bring up quite a lot of milk especially if they have taken in a large volume quickly. Slowing down the rate of milk transfer during feeds will usually reduce the volume and force of baby's vomiting. Breastfeeding mothers usually have fuller breasts in the early part of the day and the milk is likely to be taken more quickly by baby during these feeds. Some mothers with a strong letdown reflex find applying firm pressure with their hand flat across the breast during the first few minutes of the breastfeed reduces the flow enough to help baby cope with the rapid milk transfer. Expressing a little milk before the feed can reduce the force of the milk letdown so baby copes better with the feed, and vomits less.

Formula fed babies may need a slower teat, or perhaps a brand of formula which is easier to digest – this is a matter of trial and error and should be guided by a Child Health Nurse. Infant formula is made from cows' milk and vomiting may actually be caused by baby's sensitivity or allergy to cows' milk protein, which peaks during the first month of life and gradually decreases as baby's digestive system matures.

Gastro-Oesophageal Reflux Disease – GORD is a medical condition which may involve gastrointestinal, respiratory, urinary tract or ear infections, or allergic reactions. Features may include more than 5 episodes of vomiting per day, pain during feeding due to reflux of milk in the oesophagus, baby gasping or stopping breathing momentarily, and respiratory signs such as coughing and wheezing. The baby typically has poor weight gains, and is very irritable or has lengthy periods of crying.

Babies with reflux symptoms may respond to being kept upright after feeds, and trying to avoid long periods between feeds, as the milk brought up is relatively pH neutral (not acidic) for the first couple of hours after a feed. Babies less than 16 weeks of age who are only fed milk rarely have inflammation of the oesophagus (called oesophagitis or GORD), with the exception of babies who have physical abnormalities such as "floppy windpipe" or laryngomalacia. Other potential concerns such as pyloric stenosis or food protein-induced enteropathy syndrome need to be ruled out by medical tests if vomiting and crying is frequent and prolonged.

Nevertheless, research shows that two thirds of normal healthy babies can vomit regularly, and the vomiting peaks at 4 months of age. **"Silent reflux"** may be diagnosed as an explanation for frequent or prolonged crying, but there is no evidence this unsettled behaviour is caused by milk moving up and down baby's relatively short oesophagus.

It may be helpful to avoid laying the baby flat immediately after feeds. For example, slightly elevate the head of the change table mat and roll baby gently from side to side for nappy changes, rather than lifting baby's legs high. Handling baby gently and avoiding jiggling when burping baby after feeds can also reduce vomiting, and keeping clothing loose around baby's tummy, including nappies may aid comfort.

Keep baby calm before and during feeds. All babies should be kept in a smoke-free environment but tobacco smoke has been shown to significantly contribute to reflux in babies. Prescription medications may be prescribed but the bad news is studies found that medications that suppress acid production (proton pump inhibitors) are no more helpful than placebos (fake medications given during the study). Acid suppressing medications not only increase the risk of serious infections, they can predispose the baby to allergy later on, and a recent study has revealed an increased incidence of fractures in children who were given proton pump inhibitors as babies.

Reflux is worse when babies cry for prolonged periods, which affects the baby's gut because feeds become more spaced out due to the baby feeding less frequently. This causes the baby's stress levels to increase as the sympathetic nervous system is "turned up", causing altered intestinal contractions. This leads to raised abdominal pressure as baby's tummy muscles tighten during screaming, triggering reflux and vomiting. Strategies to interrupt the cycle can include taking baby for a walk outside, time-out in the shower with a parent, or trying a deep warm bath with distractions like a running tap. Carrying baby in a sling while getting on with the day's activities, or turning on some music and having a dance might help – it's a case of try this, try that during the crying periods. Take heart, it DOES pass.

COLIC

THE TERM COLIC IS USED to describe a painful condition suffered by many babies – both breastfed and formula fed, which typically occurs from about 3 weeks of age. The signs usually appear shortly after baby has been fed and settled to sleep. Baby wakes crying, may have his legs drawn up or stretched out rigidly, and his tummy may feel tight and swollen. The spasms of pain appear to be caused by wind in the lower bowel, and baby experiences the discomfort in waves with periods of calm in between periods of extreme discomfort. The term 'colic' has gone out of fashion recently and may be referred to as "unsettled periods" by some health professionals. Anyone who is experiencing this common phenomenon may feel this term barely describes what the baby and the parents are going through! Whatever you choose to call it – here are some helpful strategies to use to get through this period which I promise you, DOES usually end around 3 months of age.

Slowing down the feeds can be helpful. If bottle feeding,
use "Paced Bottle Feeding".

Source: Education.possumsonline.com

If breastfeeding, strategies to slow breastmilk transfer may also help – a Lactation Consultant can guide the mother according to her particular breast feeding situation.

If baby demonstrates feeding cues shortly after the feed appeared to be complete, feed the baby some more. These unsettled periods can also be driven by **increased hunger**. If baby is not hungry he won't feed, but if he does feed he probably needs that extra milk.

Swaddle baby after the feed, cuddle him upright (which may also help with burping), and **rock him gently** for a period after the feed before settling him to sleep. If he has a **dummy**, sucking this while settling may help to bring some wind up too. Make sure all clothing including nappies are **loose around baby's tummy** for comfort. When changing baby's nappy roll him gently from side to side rather than lifting his legs.

When unsettled or distressed, try **carrying baby** around in a sling in an upright position laid against your body. Babies need close human contact for comfort so give this, and enlist help from others when the going gets tough. Often baby will settle more readily with someone else who doesn't smell like the "milk-bar". **Go for a walk** if necessary – it will do you good too.

Another method of settling and soothing a baby with a tummy ache is to **lay him on his tummy**. This could be in a pram which you will then wheel back and forth or take for a walk, laid over Dad's arm with baby's face cradled in his hand as he rocks and walks with baby, or across an adult's lap.

Bathing baby in warm deep water, resting him on his side or tummy, or back can help make him more comfortable. Moving him slowly in the bath can help relaxation and may also help him to pass some wind. **Gentle massage** of baby's tummy in a clockwise circular motion, and cycling the legs may help him to pass the wind from his lower bowel. Some babies settle down if they are taken in the **shower** and have warm water run on their back.

If possible, try to avoid baby being exposed to excessively stimulating environments in the afternoons, eg shopping, school pick-ups, roudy visitors. Many mothers will agree their baby's colic is usually worse if they have had a really busy day out and about.

Some parents find Chiropractic and osteopathic treatments prove helpful in relieving colic. Whatever strategy you try, give it time to work – try at least 15 minutes of an activity before trying something else. When baby finally goes to sleep leave him where he has settled if possible so he gets some restful sleep and hopefully wakens in a more comfortable state.

LACTOSE OVERLOAD

WHAT CAUSES **Functional Lactose Overload** in a breastfed baby? Dr Pamela Douglas, author of "The Discontented Little Baby Book" explains it this way, which I have summarised:

"Sometimes, a breastfed baby cries a lot because of lactose overload – Lactose is the most important carbohydrate in human milk. It is dense with energy and provides 40 percent of a baby's caloric needs. Lactose has a proportionately stable concentration throughout a (breast) feed. The breast is constantly secreting all components of the milk, including fat globules ("cream"). Unlike lactose, the "cream" content in breast milk is variable, gradually increasing over the duration a feed, as the volume of milk transferred decreases. The lactase enzyme in your baby's small intestine breaks down lactose into glucose and galactose. When high loads of lactose are received the lactase enzymes can't break it all down. Undigested lactose draws water into the gut causing increased intestinal contractions. When there is lactose overload, lots of undigested lactose arrives in the colon and is fermented by bacteria, causing gases, lactic acid, and short-chain fatty acids to be released. This is when a baby might develop a bloated tummy; have acidic, frothy, explosive, frequent stools, pass lots of wind, and cry a lot. When a baby has lactose overload, her mother typically has a very generous milk supply. Although baby may be stacking on weight, there is still no reason to worry about overfeeding. Nor is there anything wrong with the milk or baby's gut enzymes. The baby's gut microbiome is likely to be altered – but it's the lactose-related fermentation and gas which cause discomfort or pain, not the accompanying (gut) dysbiosis."

So what contributes to development of lactose overload? A high milk supply, and switching sides more often than the baby needs. How is it managed? Baby is breastfed flexibly (on cue) and frequently, and returned to the same breast at least once during the series of phases of a feed. The milk in the subsequent feeds from the same breast will contain less lactose due to the smaller volume, and very likely increasing amounts of fattier milk - "cream". See a Lactation Consultant for advice about other ways of increasing baby's intake of the fattier breastmilk to help reduce the passage of high lactose milk through baby's gastrointestinal system.

AEROPHAGIA

"Proponents of surgery for (multiple) oral ties in babies with breastfeeding problems hypothesise that poor latch results in swallowed air trapped in the gut (aerophagia) which they argue worsens reflux. This hypothesis fails to consider the multiple mechanisms that underlie gastro-oesophageal reflux, including sympathetic nervous system up-regulation.

The diagnosis of Aerophagia Induced Reflux mistakes functional lactose overload for aerophagia (**Kotlow, 2016**), and exacerbates parental pressure for medical intervention" (**Scherer et al., 2013**) (**Whittingham and Douglas, 2014**). **https://www.sciencedirect.com/science/article/pii/S0266613817303467**

LATE PRE-TERM BABIES – 36-40 WEEKS

Induction of labour before the pregnancy has reached term (40 weeks) has become commonplace throughout the Western world. Maternal diagnosis of Gestational Diabetes is a key driver of this phenomenon. Mothers hoping to breastfeed their late pre-term babies can face additional challenges establishing breastfeeding because monitoring baby becomes a priority, particularly baby's blood sugar levels. Here are some practical tips to overcome the typical challenges of this situation:

Antenatal expression of colostrum from 36 weeks of pregnancy can provide some "liquid gold" colostrum for baby to have in addition to breastfeeds, avoiding the need to give formula.

Optimising **skin to skin** contact between mother and baby – a minimum of 12 hours per day has been shown to reduce the incidence of hypoglycaemia in baby. It also enhances the initiation and establishment of breastfeeding, because it enhances maternal oxytocin release.

Early feeding of colostrum in addition to breastfeeding enhances baby's establishment of normal blood glucose levels.

EXPRESSING BREASTMILK

IT HAS BECOME COMMONPLACE for mothers to express their breastmilk to give to baby by bottle, or to freeze some extra breastmilk to store for later use. Pumping, and even "double pumping" has been popularised via social media and pump manufacturers' advertisements, and embraced by mothers whose lifestyles or work commitments require baby to be separated from them for periods of time. The ability to express quickly and conveniently, even while away from baby can certainly help mothers prolong breastfeeding their babies, rather than being forced to wean baby from the breast because of returning to work.

Providing detailed guidance about expressing by pump is unfortunately beyond the scope of this book. Pumping information abounds on the internet via on-line resources. Be discerning and realistic about expressing goals, because along with the convenience there can be pitfalls as well. I offer the following suggestions to consider when you decide how to make the most of your precious expressed breastmilk.

Breastfeeding directly is the optimal way for baby to receive breastmilk as oral contact with the breast transfers pathogens from mothers skin to baby's GIT, and baby's saliva to the mother's breast via the nipple, enhancing baby's immune protection.

Frequent pumping in addition to breastfeeding can cause oversupply issues, leading to blocked ducts and mastitis. Likewise, using passive collection devices like the Haaka suction pump can cause oversupply if used excessively. It may also deprive baby of some milk during breastfeeds, potentially creating problems with weight gains.

Double pumping is not necessarily "better" than single pumping - it is a timesaver, for sure. However, if a mother is expressing to help increase her milk supply, expressing each breast individually combined with gentle breast massage and switching sides several times will usually give better results. This method simulates "switch feeding" breastfeeding technique which is an effective method of increasing milk supply when needed.

There are many pump choices available and quality and function varies. Choose carefully to ensure the pump suits your particular need, e.g. occasional use, regular use, or expressing periodically to establish or increase milk production.

If the reason for expressing is to supply breastmilk for a prematurely born baby, hiring a hospital grade pump for use at home is recommended for best results during this critical period. Further information about optimising breastmilk expression for a premature baby: **https://med.stanford.edu/ newborns/professional-education/breastfeeding/maximizing-milk-production.html**

Most modern breast pumps now feature "closed filtration" systems, which means milk cannot be accidentally transferred to the pump via the tubing creating a potential pathogen hazard. Closed filtration system pumps can therefore be loaned or sold between mothers safely, however purchase of new tubing is recommended. The older Medela personal use pumps (eg Swing) did not have closed filtration systems and are intended for single person use only.

Choose a pump with good range of variability of suction **strength** settings. Settings for **frequency** of suction may be less variable – increased variability of settings aids comfort and safety of use. I have seen several really nasty wounds inflicted by cheap pumps when mothers have had suction strength turned up high, trying to express more effectively. With breast pumps you get what you pay for.

Make sure the flange size and shape suits the breast and nipple size and shape. Incorrectly fitted flanges can cause injuries and impair effective milk transfer. If friction is a problem even with a correctly fitted flange, placing a little coconut oil inside the nipple barrel can improve comfort and function.

Be aware expressing regularly can be both reassuring and worrisome. Mothers naturally take note of the volumes they are collecting and can become very focussed on meeting certain target amounts at each expressing session. Using "feeding or expressing apps" can be helpful to record volumes yielded, but can also be misleading if the app information dominates the mother's focus, rather than observing her baby's cues and responses. Breastmilk production naturally varies enormously at different times of the day or night, and from day to day influenced by a variety of factors, many of which are beyond the mother's control.

BREAST SURGERY

WOMEN WHO HAVE HAD breast surgeries (breast reduction, breast implants, nipple surgery) should seek advice from an IBCLC (Lactation Consultant). Breast implants can contribute to serious engorgement in the early days after birth, and breast reduction surgery can impact a mother's ability to achieve a full supply. Expert guidance from a Lactation Consultant can address these issues and potentially help mothers achieve their breastfeeding goals.

TOPIC 6
NAPPY TIME (DIAPERS)

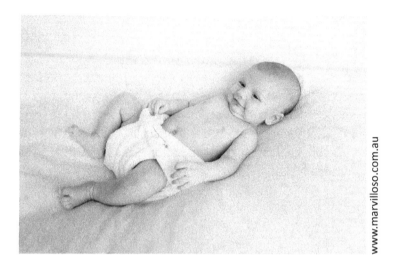

www.marvilloso.com.au

CARING FOR YOUR BABY'S HYGIENE and skin are probably the most basic skills a parent must learn from Day 1 of baby's life. Newborn babies are capable of astonishing output in their nappies from birth as the sticky black meconium begins to move through their gastro-intestinal tract (GIT) in response to suckling the Mother's breast, and receiving the nutritive and protective colostrum which also has natural laxative properties.

I have observed hundreds of new Mums and Dads tackle their first meconium poo nappy and heard some really funny responses over the years to this task.   So far I've never heard a new parent say – "No, I just can't do it" because they all know this is part of the deal, and they have to approach nappytime with diligence and humour. Thankfully most Dads are closely involved in baby's care these days, including changing nappies. I have already provided a guide to setting up you change table in **Topic 1 – What do we really need?** Your change table is likely to be the most frequently used item of equipment in your nursery for the next couple of years, so here is a summary of the most important points and suggestions to help you manage this repetitive but also rewarding task as you care for your new baby.

NAPPY CHANGE STATION

YOU NEED TO SET UP a 'change station' before baby is born so it is all ready to go as this is sure to be one of the first jobs you will need to do when you get home! You could use a change pad on top of a chest of drawers or a table or a bench which is stable and easily accessible, or you may buy or borrow a purpose built change table with a change pad or mat. It needs to be waterproof and easy to clean as this will be the most frequently used item in your home for about a year.

A clean towel or cloth nappy folded on the surface makes it more comfortable for baby. I recommend parents avoid using cleansing products including nappy wipes on their newborn baby's delicate skin. Using water (which can be warm) and cotton balls or Chux wipes to clean baby's bottom is cheap and safe and more comfortable for baby than cold nappy wipes, which are all impregnated with chemicals of some kind. Use Chux or a towelling washer to dry baby's skin after cleansing.

Nappy Wipes – these are handy to use when you are out and water is not available to cleanse baby's bottom however using them for every nappy change can mean baby's delicate bottom is frequently exposed to chemicals of some type, even though claims of "gentle and organic" appear reassuring. Baby's skin is very thin and receptive to any applied chemicals. **"Water Wipes"** are guaranteed to only contain water and no chemicals. There are a number of health concerns associated with chemical-laden commercial nappy wipes.

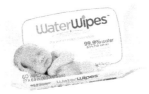

A simple zinc and castor oil nappy cream can be used AFTER cleansing if any nappy rashes appear. Baby talcum powder is not recommended as it clogs the skin and particles can be breathed in by baby. Cotton wool balls and plain water are ideal for cleansing baby's face, eyes and ears as well as nappy area – watch the New Baby 101 **video "How to Bath Baby"** to see a demonstration of cleansing baby's eyes and face. A thermos to hold some warm water is a handy addition to the cleansing items near the change station if there is not a tap nearby.

Two packets of 20 NEWBORN size disposable nappies will get you started. If you are interested in using cloth nappies, flannelette nappy squares can be folded smaller and are less bulky than towelling nappies on newborns. There are also many ready-made fabric nappies with Velcro fastenings available which are comfortable for baby, but these take longer to dry after washing than flannelette nappies. Whichever nappy option you choose, it is advisable to give baby some "nappy-off time" each day to allow baby's skin to 'breathe'.

You will need a rubbish bin with a lid, and a basket for baby's soiled clothes and wraps near the change station. A month's supply of flannelette nappies from a nappy wash service is a great present to have on your baby shower list. **Watch New Baby 101 "How to change a baby's nappy" video**

DIFFERENCES YOU NEED TO KNOW ABOUT BOYS AND GIRLS

A BABY BOY HAS an intact penis which nature has designed perfectly. The glans in enclosed in the foreskin which protects the sensitive tissue and allows it to function normally, passing urine and sometimes having little erections which are normal too, and provides a warning to parents that the spout is about to function! The foreskin should be left alone and just gently washed in the bath and cleansed as needed with plain water using a cotton ball. It is painful and unnecessary to retract the foreskin of little boys. They will discover that pleasure when they are 3 or 4 years old, and will naturally explore their own anatomy finding out what is comfortable and pleasurable and what is not. In the meantime the baby boy's penis belongs to him and decisions about whether to surgically change the appearance and function of his penis should also be his.

Circumcision of baby's boys is discouraged by health professionals around the world. This matter is discussed in more detail in **Topic 2 – Early Decisions**, and you can view **www.birthjourney.com** for more information.

Complications after infant circumcision surgery can be very serious and even fatal. If circumcision is performed on a baby boy it is essential to follow the medical advice provided about surgical dressings and careful cleansing of the wound until it is completely healed. Babies should be given regular oral pain relief medication for at least a week and if any signs of infection appear medical care must be sought immediately.

Baby girls just need their external vulva gently cleansed of wee and poo using plain water and cotton balls. It is important to always cleanse a baby girl's bottom in a stroking motion from <u>front to back</u>. An upward motion from back to front could transfer poo from the rectum to the vagina and urethra and cause bacterial contamination and potential infection of those delicate areas. A front to back action will ensure this can't happen.

Newborn baby girls often have a mucousy discharge from the vagina, which may also be blood stained or just blood (called 'frank blood"). Although this may be disturbing to the parents it is a normal occurrence due to the flood of hormones which occurs in the baby girl's body. Sometimes the flow of mucous or blood from the baby girl's vagina can be quite profuse and continue for several weeks. This is normal and will not harm the baby. Parents should just cleanse the nappy area as described before. The infantile menses will settle down over time.

Baby girls sometimes have little skin tags which protrude from the labia or vagina. These do not usually cause problems and gradually shrink and recede out of view as the baby grows. Both baby girls and baby boys may also have swollen breasts caused by the same surge of hormones. Occasionally a waxy milk like substance may ooze from the breasts called "witches milk". This is of no concern and the swollen little breasts should be left alone to recede naturally. If the breasts become inflamed and red medical attention should be sought, as baby may need treatment with antibiotics.

POOS AND WEES

COPIOUS AMOUNTS OF sticky black meconium are passed by the newborn in the first day or two of life. Then the colour begins to change to brownish (called "transitional stools") and when baby is digesting milk the poo changes to a mustardy yellow with a soft runny consistency in breastfed babies, and a more formed light brown stool in formula-fed babies. Your baby's wees and poos are a good guide to how the baby's feeding is going.

Newborn babies are born a bit water-logged, and the urine they pass in the early days is a response to this natural fluid release rather than a reflection of the amount of colostrum they have taken during breastfeeds. On Day 1 of life we expect one wee, on Day 2 of life we expect 2 wees, and from Day 3 of life onwards we expect 3 or more wees. By Day 3 the wees should be making the disposable nappy quite heavy.

 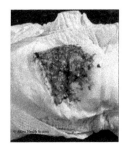 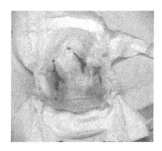

Meconium   **Breastmilk stools**   **Urates in urine**

Baby boys and girls may also pass **urates** in their nappies with urine. This appears as a pinkish/orange tinted spot in the wet nappy. Parents are often alarmed at this pink spot in baby's wet nappy, thinking it is blood. These are crystals expelled by the kidneys as they are kick-starting their function, and are of no concern in newborn babies. If urates appear in an older baby's nappy it is NOT normal. In these early days it can be difficult to decide whether there is a wee and a poo, or just a poo in each nappy. Placing a couple of cotton balls inside the nappy near the penis of a baby boy, or further back and central in the nappy of a baby girl can be helpful to determine when baby has done a wee. Otherwise it can be difficult to be sure by just feeling a disposable nappy in the first few days. As mentioned before, the baby's output – the wees and the poos are a useful guide to how much milk baby is taking during breastfeeds.

The expected output of a well newborn from Day 3-4 onwards is 6-8 nappies per day, and 3 or more of these should be poos. If a breastfed baby is producing 2 or less poos in each 24 hours from day 3 onwards, this is the first indication that the volume of breastmilk being transferred to baby may be insufficient. Many parents are tricked by the fact that baby continues to do wees. It is the poo which gives the real indication of milk transfer, not the urine output. If a parent is concerned that their newborn baby is not producing sufficient wees and poos they should take baby to be checked by a Child Health Nurse, Lactation Consultant or GP.

Colour of Poo – baby's poo colour may vary as she grows, particularly if breastfed. Baby's poo may look green-ish if the mother has eaten an abundance of green foods or is taking iron supplements. Green frothy poo can indicate baby is digesting rapidly, and baby may also be gassy and uncomfortable/crying often. Lactose overload may be the cause – refer to page 49 for more information. Green mucousy poo may indicate baby is unwell, or is sensitive to Cow's Milk Protein (CMP), which requires review by a GP or Paediatrician.

UMBILICAL CORD CARE

NAPPY CHANGE TIME IS the ideal opportunity to care for baby's umbilical cord stump. Baby may still have the cord clamp in place when he is discharged home from hospital. Ensure the clamp is always positioned outside the nappy. This will be more comfortable for baby and also assist the umbilical cord to dry out which is necessary to enable it to fall off, and for the umbilical base to heal. This area should be gently cleansed with plain water and a cotton ball or cotton tip at each nappy change. Keeping this area clean and dry will assist it to heal. It is not necessary or recommended to apply any other products (eg. methylated spirits, antiseptic creams or powders, or betadine solution) to the umbilical stump for cleansing or to enhance healing. These products will in fact slow separation and healing of the umbilical stump. If the area becomes red have it checked by your Midwife or Child Health Nurse. The stump will naturally become a bit smelly as it dries up and becomes ready to fall off. When the stump has separated continue to cleanse the umbilicus base with water and a cotton ball at each nappy change and the area should heal within a few days.

TYPES OF NAPPIES

SIMPLY STATED – the choice is **Disposable or Reusable.** Convenience, cost and environmental impact are the key issues to consider. The range of options within the two broad categories is vast and a matter of discussion and debate amongst parents. A typical baby will use 6 to 7000 nappies until fully toilet trained. Here are some considerations –

Convenience – there is no doubt disposable nappies are convenient to use, especially in the early months of baby's life when frequent nappy changes are necessary, coinciding with frequent feeds.

Cost – This factor becomes a reality when new parents realise how quickly the bottom of the nappy packet or box appears in the first few months of baby's life. Once parents find which nappy serves them best, buying in bulk is definitely advisable and keeping a close watch on 'specials' becomes a regular focus of shopping trips. Buying disposable nappies can easily consume over $100 per month or $1200 per year. Baby is likely to be in nappies for about 2 years and although the frequency of changes reduces as they grow, the bigger nappies and pull ups are more expensive.

If you're thinking about that last point, here are some key ideas to keep in mind:
- The upfront cost of cloth nappies can be quite high but decreases in cost per wear with each child
- The cheapest cloth option is terry towelling at $1 to $2 per nappy, but they can be tricky to get used to – see the New Baby 101 video for folding options!
- Modern cloth nappies range from about $7 to $35, which means they're initially more expensive
- Disposables are often more convenient and start at just 16 cents per nappy up to over $1 each for some eco-friendly brands
- Baby wipes and creams can be a hidden cost, so try to factor them in as well

Environmental issues should certainly be factored into this decision. New parents quickly realise how much space their newborn's used nappies take up in their wheelie bin each week, and the impact of disposable nappies on landfill is enormous.

Traditional cloth nappy squares still offer a cost effective and environmentally friendly option. Purchased in packs of 6 or 12, flannelette or towelling fabric nappy squares are simple to wash and dry, and can be folded in a variety of ways to suit boy or girl babies of all ages. They double as convenient spill catchers and change table cover savers. These nappies will often last well enough to serve two or more babies, and make great cleaning cloths for years to come after that! To see 5 ways to fold cloth nappies view the New Baby 101 **video "How to fold a Traditional Cloth Nappy/diaper".**

Remember also that baby has a nappy on almost 24/7 for the first two or three years of his life! This is a long time to be encased in plastic so "nappy off time" is a really important daily routine to adopt to protect your baby's skin integrity and comfort. Watch the **New Baby 101 video "How to change baby's nappy/diaper" https://youtu.be/-u42vEMjg40** to see a demonstration of how to fold and put on a comfortable flannelette **cloth nappy which does not need pins** which is an easy alternative for newborns having a few hours break from plastic covered disposable nappies/diapers.

CHOICE magazine has done extensive trials over many years on disposable and reusable/cloth nappies and have found that there has been a shift in parents' nappy preferences in recent years. Where 95% previously used disposable nappies, one in five of trialists in their most recent study were using cloth nappies or a mix of cloth and disposable, and an on-line poll showed 40% of respondents preferred cloth nappies. For all the results of CHOICE's trials and parents' feedback about disposable nappies and Modern Cloth nappies visit: **http://www.choice.com.au/reviews-and-tests/babies-and-kids**

Research conducted by the University of Queensland showed that home-washed reusable nappies, washed in cold water in a front-loading washing machine and line dried, are the most environmentally friendly option. ABC News also "crunched the numbers" in 2020 and interviewed some parents to discuss the pro's and con's – scan the QR code below:

NAPPY/DIAPER RASH

MOST BABIES WILL develop a nappy rash at some time in their lives however there are some strategies which will help avoid this happening, and speed up healing if nappy rash does occur. Baby's nappy should be changed as soon as it is wet or pooey, as the urine and poo can irritate baby's skin even if the nappy is very absorbent.

If a breastfeeding Mum or baby have been on antibiotics baby's poo can change in consistency and odour, and also be more irritating to baby's skin. Avoid using baby wipes on irritated skin as they WILL sting and potentially make the rash worse. Use plain water to cleanse baby's bottom with cotton balls which are gentler than most fabrics. Dry the skin by gently dabbing with a soft facewasher, and apply a nappy cream - Zinc and castor oil based creams provide a good barrier. **Bepanthen** cream has been proven by research to aid healing of nappy rashes. Allowing baby to have 'nappy off time" every day will also aid healing.

If baby has **oral thrush** (a white plaque visible on baby's tongue and inside the cheeks which cannot be scraped off easily) baby may also get thrush in the nappy area – seen as a raised red rash which will require treatment with an antifungal cream. Visit your Child Health Nurse for advice about types of rashes, and if a baby's nappy rash does not respond quickly to the basic care as described, a doctor should be consulted for assessment and treatment.

If a breastfed baby does have thrush both the baby and the mother need to be treated simultaneously.

TOPIC 7
Bathtime

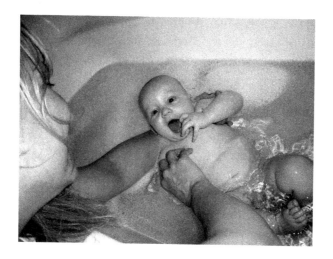

THERE ARE SOME BASIC SAFE PRACTICES to adhere to when bathing your baby, but there is only **one rule – NEVER leave your baby unattended in water, at any age.** Bathing a newborn can be a bit scarey for new parents. In the early weeks bathing often seems to take a long time with baby getting tired and unhappy in the process. This can be avoided by planning baby's bath AFTER a feed (or after the first phase of a feed) rather than the traditional regime of bathing baby before being fed. I think the rationale for feeding baby AFTER a bath was in case it made baby vomit if they had just been fed. Actually this is not a big deal, even if baby does spit up some milk it's easy to clean up at bathtime! If baby spends the whole bathtime crying miserably due to hunger he certainly is not going to enjoy his bath, and he may also be so tired from crying he won't feed well anyway.

Baby does not need to be bathed every day – it can be an alternate days' job. Washing baby's face, hands and bottom (in that order) can be done instead if it's not convenient to do a bath. You can also take baby into the shower instead of bathing him in the traditional way – this is a good job for Dad but Mum needs to be on hand to take baby out to dry and dress him. There are no rules - do what works for you and find what your baby enjoys. Some time in the shower can be a great settling strategy if baby is overtired or unsettled.

To give baby a traditional bath you can use a baby bath, or a clean basin, sink or laundry trough. Some baby baths come with a stand and an outlet hose to make emptying easier. You may be able to borrow a baby bath from a friend as they tend to be used for the first few months and then baby graduates to being bathed in the adult size bath. Placing a baby bath into your adult bath and using it there can make filling and emptying the baby bath easier. If Mum has had a caesarean section a full baby bath is too heavy for her to lift or carry. A baby bath thermometer is an inexpensive, handy and reassuring item to have for checking the bath water temperature which should be around 37C. **Watch the New Baby 101 video "<u>How to Bath Your Baby</u>".**

HERE IS A BASIC GUIDE FOR BATHING BABY

ONE PIECE OF ADVICE - remember the nappy is the **last** thing to come **off** and the **first** thing to go on!

Choose a location where you can provide a warm, draft free environment. This may be your kitchen or bathroom, but it needs to be near water taps and a sink for draining the bath water.

Get everything you are going to need ready before bathtime.
You will need:
Two soft clean towels
Cotton balls
Face washer
Full set of baby clothes and nappy
Nappy cream if needed
Baby wash if you are using it on baby's hair.
Baby bath water thermometer
Spread the towels ready to use, and have everything else within easy reach but not where they could get wet. (Beware of baby boy's ability to wee a distance and wet fresh clothes!)

Fill the bath with warm water. Measure the temperature and allow it to be a little above 37 degrees Celsius as it will cool while you undress baby. Recheck the temperature with you're your elbow before putting baby into the bath. It should be comfortably warm, never hot. If your newborn's skin is very dry and peeling a teaspoon of olive oil in the bathwater will moisturise baby's skin without clogging the skin pores.

Lay baby on one of the towels and undress her, all except her nappy.
Wrap her in the towel and using warm wet cotton balls, wash her face.
When cleansing her eyes, gently stroke a cotton ball from the inside of one eye to the outside, and discard it. Do the same with the other eye with and a new wet cotton ball, and discard. Use wet cotton balls to clean her ears and neck, and under her chin.

You can wash her head now, or at the end of the bath. If the environment is cool, leave washing her head and hair until last so she does not lose too much body heat during the bath time. To wash her head, wrap her firmly in the towel and hold her securely under your arm with her head positioned over the bath, facing upwards looking at you. Use a facewasher to wet her head, avoiding water running on her face. If using some baby bath solution for her hair put a little onto the facewasher and lightly lather her head, then rinse it using the face washer.

* Handy hint for newborns with blood stuck in their hair – put a teaspoon of olive oil and a dob of baby bath solution in the palm of your hand, mix them, and then apply them to the bloody sections on baby's head before the bath. When cleansing baby's head the old blood will wash out without rubbing hard on baby's tender scalp.

Return baby to beside the bath and dry her head if it is wet. Now take off her nappy. Cleanse any poo which you may find there before putting her into the water.

Hold baby behind the shoulders, grasping the shoulder and arm furthest from you, and also grasp both baby's feet. Lift baby and place her gently into the bath, letting go of her feet but continue holding onto the shoulder and arm securely as you swish the water with your opposite hand and bathe her using the facecloth. Bathe the upper body first, working you're your way downwards towards her bottom, legs and feet. Pay attention to cleanse in the folds of her groin, and sit her forward to bathe her back. When washing a baby girl's bottom, always cleanse from the front to the back. Be gentle with baby boy's genitals, and never move the foreskin back to cleanse it.

Help baby to relax by talking to her about what you are doing together. A folded hand towel or muslin wrap in the bottom of the bath water can make the base more comfortable for baby. If baby really hates being uncovered in the bathwater, place a clean wet face washer over her chest and legs so she feels more covered and secure. You can even put baby into the water in a muslin wrap if she is unhappy about being naked in the bath. These are all strategies which may help baby feel more secure when being bathed. There are also little stands and seats which can be used in the bath, but these are more for parents' security than for baby's. Be careful when learning how to use these gadgets, and never leave baby unattended no matter now secure the little seat may appear.

Don't leave baby in the water too long as it will cool quickly. When she's done lift her the same way you put her in, and lay her on the dry towel, wrapping her quickly. Dry her hair and head first. Then unwrap her legs and bottom to dry her thoroughly, then put on the nappy. Finish drying baby's upper body and face, and roll her over onto her tummy to dry her back and hair again. When she is nice and dry, put on her singlet, then her clothes. Don't use talcum powder on baby – it clogs the pores and can also be inhaled by baby as it is dusted on. If you REALLY want to put some on for that lovely freshly bathed scent, just dust a little onto the back of her singlet before dressing her. Avoid using creams and lotions on baby's skin as they can clog the pores and irritate the skin – even if they are 'gentle' or 'organic' or other claims made by product manufacturers.

Cutting baby's fingernails – The easiest time to cut baby's fingernails is after a bath, when she is asleep. You can use baby nail clippers, but the method I prefer is to use little nail scissors with rounded ends for baby. You make a tiny snip at the corner of the long finger nail, then peel it off. This method does not leave any sharp corners on the nails.

You can also use a fine emery board very gently on baby's nails if you wish. Some parents prefer to bite their baby's finger nails instead of cutting them

Cradle Cap is a scaly, crusty area of skin which develops on baby's scalp, and often over the forehead as well. Washing baby's hair each time he is bathed and using a soft baby brush on his scalp daily will help prevent cradle cap.

A traditional remedy is to rub a little olive oil into the crusty areas an hour or so before baby is bathed, then wash the areas with plain water, or with a gentle soap free wash such as **Moo Goo Milk Wash. Moo Goo Scalp Cream** is safe and effective for treatment of Cradle Cap. If Cradle Cap or other flaky skin problems persists ask your Child Health Nurse to assess baby's skin condition. Excessive crustiness of baby's scalp and forehead can be a sign of an allergy related to baby's feeding. Seek medical advice if this occurs.

BABY'S SKIN

MOST PARENTS WORRY ABOUT SPOTS AND RASHES with pin-head sized pimples which appear on baby's skin but these are usually harmless and normal variations and responses to baby's skin adjusting to the different environment to the womb. Newborn babies may take a few days to lose that 'crumpled' appearance, and often have a flat nose, lumps on their head, puffy eyes and red blotches on their face and body. Their whole body often looks very red and ruddy (called **plethoric**) and their hands and feet usually look blue-ish grey (called **acrocyanosis**) – this is normal and baby's skin colour will adjust in a few days. It is NOT normal for baby to look blue-ish grey on the face or body. This would indicate baby is oxygen-deprived and needs immediate assessment of breathing and urgent medical attention.

Some babies may also have bruises from the birth process, a wound on their scalp from a probe installed to monitor their heartbeat during labour, or marks or bruises from vacuum cups or forceps. All of these will fade quite quickly, except for a **cephalhaematoma** (collection of blood forming a lump on baby's scalp) which can take many weeks or even months to fully disappear. Baby is more prone to **JAUNDICE** if bruising has occurred (see **Topic 5**). Baby's skin may also look slightly mottled, especially if he is cool. Although usually normal, mottled skin can also be an indication baby is unwell so take baby's temperature and if it is elevated you should see a doctor as soon as possible. You do not need to take baby's temperature routinely when he is healthy, only if he feels hot to touch or is unwell.

BABY'S FACE AND HEAD

BABY MAY HAVE tiny white-ish pimple-like dots across her nose called **MILIA**. These are normal and should not be squeezed or treated. They disappear naturally after a few weeks. Baby may also have a red mark across his upper eyelids, forehead or back of the neck. Called "**Stork Beak or Stork Bite Marks**", these are caused by a group of blood vessels close to the surface of the skin. They are very common particularly in fair skinned babies and usually fade by about two years of age. Parents may notice these 'birth marks' look brighter red when baby is upset. When faded in older children, they reappear when the child is angry or crying. They do not require any treatment of any kind.

A newborn baby's head shape can vary enormously dependent on his journey from the womb. Baby's head is designed to change shape to fit through the mother's pelvis and birth canal, so this moulding process can result in baby having a long shaped cone-head, a lop-sided head, or a very flat shape to the top of his head if baby has been in the breech position. Fortunately baby's head shape adjusts very quickly once the birth is completed. Baby's face may appear to be lop-sided (asymmetrical) too, and usually adjusts over the following weeks as baby uses his facial muscles and jaw to feed. It is important to alternate which side baby is facing when he is laid on his back to sleep to avoid baby's head becoming flat at the back called "plagiocephaly".

BABY'S EYES

A BABY MAY LOOK CROSS-EYED at times when they are endeavouring to focus, but this common, and not of any concern. Eye co-ordination develops as baby grows. A red bloodspot may be seen in baby's eye (called a **subconjuctival haemorrhage**) when a small blood vessel has burst during the birth. Although it looks nasty it does not cause baby any pain or harm, and the blood will be reabsorbed in 7-10 days and disappear.

The **sclera** or whites of baby's eyes may have a blue-ish tint, or in a jaundiced baby they may be quite yellow-looking. This will disappear as the jaundice resolves. Baby's tear ducts don't function to produce tears until she is about 1 month old, and the tear ducts may need gentle massage and cleansing if they become blocked.

Sticky eyes are common in newborns and easily treated with frequent cleansing with cooled boiled water and cotton balls using the method as demonstrated in the **video: "How to Bath Your Baby"**. Putting drops of breastmilk in the eyes each time baby is settling to sleep will often clear the problem in a day or so. If this does not resolve quickly baby may need eye ointment prescribed by the doctor.

HOW TO TAKE BABY'S TEMPERATURE –

PLACE THE TIP OF a digital thermometer under baby's arm directly against the skin, with a skinfold surrounding the tip of the thermometer. Leave the thermometer in place until it alarms. Read and write down the temperature and the time it was taken. Normal temperature range is from 36.5 to 37.5 degrees Celsius (97.7 – 99.5 F). If baby is hot take off a layer of clothing or wraps. Take the baby's temperature again after 30 minutes and compare the readings. If baby's temperature remains elevated seek medical attention.

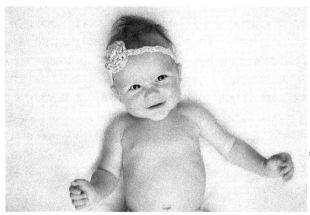

www.marvilloso.com.au

TOPIC 8
Bedtime - Sleep and Settling

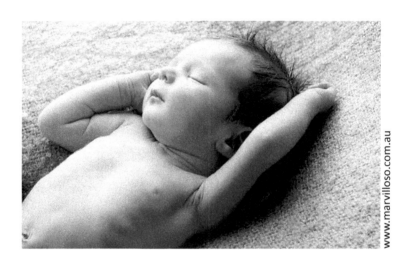

www.marvilloso.com.au

THIS TOPIC IS OFTEN DISCUSSED at length by parents and health experts and is probably the most controversial baby-care issue to address. It has become a major focus among many parents in the western world, while parents in other countries hardly ever discuss their baby's sleep patterns or their bedtime practices.   This book covers the first three months of baby's life so the information contained in this topic relates specifically to young babies.

Once new parents understand **how** babies sleep they will realise it is unnatural and unrealistic to try to impose rigid sleep and feed routines on young babies.   Consider the animal kingdom. All animals feed and sleep and play. Over thousands of years they have evolved to keep their babies close to them from birth, and to feed them whenever they indicate that need. This is an instinctive protective behaviour to ensure the survival of the species. The mother is totally focussed on guarding her baby from predators and danger, and the baby is 'hardwired' to stay close to its mother at all times.

Humans have also evolved over many thousands of years and in spite of very recent technological developments the biological foundations of conception, birth and nurture of babies are still exquisitely embedded in human instincts. Our babies are "hardwired" to be close to their mothers and to demonstrate their needs with non-verbal signals which attentive parents recognise and respond to accordingly. Parents are swimming against the tide of human DNA when they try to manipulate their baby's natural instinctive behaviours to fit the western world's demands about feeding and sleep. Yes, we live in a modern sophisticated environment, but a human's biological functioning is the same as it was a hundred years ago, or a thousand years ago, or more.

Expectations regarding baby's sleep can be the source of great anxiety for parents if they believe their baby is not sleeping 'well' or 'enough'. Understanding how variable baby's sleep patterns are from baby to baby, and from week to week according to individual feeding, growth and developmental stages can relieve parents' concerns, and free them to 'go with the flow' of their baby's individual needs.

Parents will learn how to interpret their baby's needs by closely observing baby's facial expressions and movements. By learning to read baby's signals you will understand her various **awake and sleep states** – yes, there are more than two! When awake, babies can be quiet alert, active alert or crying which is their principal means of communicating a need. Drowsiness leads to sleep. Baby's sleep states transition between active sleep and quiet sleep. Drowsiness upon waking transitions to the quiet alert state often combined with feeding cues – the perfect time to feed baby. Young babies often move from state to state quickly so parents who respond to baby's changing cues swiftly are likely to encounter fewer feeding and sleep problems.

As the early weeks of baby's life unfolds a pattern emerges, and the new parents can begin to relax and embrace their new life-style. This does not mean baby is dictating the terms of existence forever after. It means the parents are meeting their baby's needs responsibly and sensitively as their new family becomes a cohesive functioning unit. I will describe the awake and sleep states in a little more detail as understanding this is fundamental to interpreting your baby's life rhythm, which will ultimately make life more enjoyable for all of you.

AWAKE STATES

DROWSINESS – When baby is in a drowsy state his body movements will be smooth and his eyelids will look heavy as they open and close when he is waking from sleep. He may yawn and drift in and out of sleep as he is wakening. He may startle at sounds or sudden movements. Drowsiness will appear much the same when he is drifting from an awake state to a sleep state.

Quiet Alert - baby will be attentive and absorbed in whoever or whatever is within his view. He may respond with facial movements and coo-ing mouth and voice sounds. The quiet alert state is ideal for interacting with your baby with facial expressions, words and song and waiting for his responses.

Active Alert – baby will be clearly aware of movement and sound around her, turning her head to look at toys or other stimuli. She may respond with body movements and vocal sounds, and engage in play with toys or pictures, especially faces. If and when she has had enough she will begin to fuss, and be more sensitive to noises. She may look away from you. She is letting you know she is ready for a change of pace, and it is wise to back-off with the stimulation, removing her to a quieter environment if necessary.

Crying – is baby's way of communicating she needs something, or soothing. As parents become more tuned-in to their baby's pre-crying signs they will be able to avert situations where baby really can't cope and cries for relief or comfort. Baby will need to be comforted by being held close and verbally reassured that all is well and you are nearby. Not responding to a baby's cry for comfort will add to baby's distress. Conversely, responding to baby's **early** cues day and night will help baby to develop a sense of trust in his world and form a secure attachment to you. Babies learn 'self regulation' by calming down after being distressed.

SLEEP STATES

ACTIVE SLEEP - When baby calms down and his needs of comfort (eg. nappy change) and hunger are met, a state of drowsiness will follow. Baby will drift into an Active Sleep state, often stirring frequently with jerky startle movements, and flickering eyelids as baby is in REM (Rapid Eye Movement) sleep. It can be helpful to stay with baby with your hands resting firmly on him as he **settles in his bed**. He will feel secure, like he is still being held, as he moves from Active Sleep into **Quiet Sleep**. You will feel baby 'sink' gently away from your hands as he relaxes into a deeper sleep state. His breathing rate will be regular and deep, his face will be still. Now is the time to lift your hands quietly and move away. Baby may make sucking movements, or startle briefly during Quiet Sleep, but he does not fully waken so allow him time to return to sleep.

Babies have short sleep cycles compared to adults, moving frequently between active and quiet sleep states. Adult sleep cycles are about 90 minutes long, while up to about 3 months of age baby's sleep cycle lasts about 45 minutes - divided into about 25 minutes of active sleep, followed by 20 minutes of quiet sleep. Babies stir frequently between sleep states. These arousals are believed to be part of their inbuilt survival mechanism protecting them from SIDS. Baby's sleep patterns alter as they progress through developmental changes and growth spurts, so it is a sign of normal growth for baby to go through periods of sleeping well and being less settled at other times.

TIRED SIGNS

JUST AS BABIES SIGNAL TO THEIR PARENTS that they are hungry by showing "feeding cues", they also show "tired signs" when they need to sleep. Parents will quickly learn to recognise and respond to their young baby's signs of tiring, such as jerky arm movements and yawning, frowning, fussing, and looking away from stimulating toys or faces. An overtired baby may find it difficult to go to sleep even though rest is what they desperately need. View the New Baby 101 **video "How To Swaddle Your Baby"** to see baby William demonstrating 'tired signs'.

A newborn baby will become tired when they have been awake for an hour or more - including the time taken for feeding. Their arms become tense, and they may arch backwards when being held. Fussing turns to crying and when very overtired they may 'lose the plot' making it difficult to calm down. Cuddling baby close, and offering a clean finger to suck, the breast or a dummy can break the crying cycle. Young babies often need another breast feed to calm down, and drift off to sleep.

I emphasise the importance of responding to baby's early feeding cues for best results, and the message about tired signs is similar. Respond to baby's **early tired signs** by preparing baby for comfort and sleep. This may mean moving baby away from a stimulating environment to a quieter zone, changing baby's nappy if needed, cuddling baby close and reassuring baby in a relaxed soothing voice, and offering a feed if baby seems hungry. Baby can then be swaddled and either cuddled until drowsy or asleep, or placed gently in his bed to drift off to sleep.

If baby does not settle easily stay with him, with your hands resting on him for reassurance so he feels he is still being held. Patting gently on his bottom often helps baby to relax. Sometimes baby will settle more easily laid on his side. This is fine if you are with him. He can be gently moved onto his back when he is asleep, but he CAN be settled on his side if he prefers it.

Babies do not need to be taught to "self sooth" to go to sleep ie. put themselves to sleep without your help. Dr Pamela Douglas advises: "Various factors, such as whether the baby is fed breast milk or formula, where the baby sleeps, and how quickly parents respond to their baby's cries, interact with the biological regulation of sleep...If parents simply remove obstacles to healthy sleep, and then proceed to enjoy the day, the baby's sleep will look after itself with minimal effort on the parents' part". Source: *"The Discontented Little Baby"* P143

STILL HUNGRY?

IF BABY DOES NOT SETTLE when you expect him to, it is likely he actually needs to be fed some more. Don't ignore feeding cues when your plan is to settle baby to sleep. Believe me, the need to feed will over-rule your best efforts to settle him. If in doubt, offer another feed. This will save you time and energy in the long run, and will not "spoil" or overfeed baby. Young babies under 3 months old need feeds in multiple instalments. They often need more food after a bowel movement and clean up to feel satisfied again and ready to sleep. Follow baby's cues and the bliss of dreamland will soon be yours.

WHY DOES A BREASTFEED PROMOTE SLEEP?

BABY FALLING ASLEEP WHILE BREASTFEEDING is biologically normal. Breastfeeding stimulates the release of the hormone cholecystokinin (CCK) which has a sedating effect on both the mother and the baby. The natural relaxation effect of breastfeeding enhances bonding between mother and baby, and skin to skin contact stimulates release of another hormone, oxytocin, often called the hormone of love. Oxytocin causes feelings of maternal love in the mother and calm wellbeing in baby.

The CCK released by the breastfeeding mother enhances the depth of her sleep when she goes back to bed after a night feed, so the quality of sleep she experiences helps her to feel less fatigued in the daytime compared to a mother who formula feeds her baby. The levels of Prolactin (the Mother's milk-making hormone) are naturally higher at night time so night feeds assist with establishment and maintenance of an adequate breast milk supply for her growing baby.

NIGHT AND DAY

WHEN BABY WAS INSIDE HIS MOTHER'S WOMB he was influenced by her physical movements and activities such as eating and sleeping, but he was not affected by light and dark, night and day. In this protected environment baby was surrounded by warm water, securely tucked in, consistently nurtured by his mother's blood supply, and gently rocked around and soothed by his mother's daily physical activities and the sounds of her voice and her body's functions.

When a baby is born he must adapt to his new world outside of the womb. Light, sound, touch, pain, clothing, poos and wees, sucking, swallowing and breathing are all new experiences for baby. Once on the outside, baby will continue to be comforted by what is most familiar to him. **Warmth** – close to his mother's body in skin to skin contact. **Security** – contained in soft wraps and held in loving arms. **Nurture** – receiving food as frequently as he seeks it – warm, nutritious and sweet breastmilk and the delicious comfort of suckling mother's breast. **Movement and soft sounds** – gentle rocking and swaying simulating mother's movements as she went about her day whilst pregnant, and the soft vibrations and sounds of her voice. It should not be surprising that baby takes some time to adapt to sleeping in a place away from his mother, and needs to revisit the familiar comforts often for reassurance that all is well in this wide strange world.

Young babies are dominated by their needs for food, comfort and sleep rather than the environmental stimuli of light and dark, day and night. Circadian rhythms dictate our internal body clocks which influence energy levels, sleep patterns and moods. Two main hormones control circadian rhythms and are influenced by the light of day and the darkness of night. Cortisol is the stimulating "get going in the morning" hormone, and the other hormone Melatonin peaks in the evening in response to reducing light, helping the body "wind down" in preparation for sleep. Newborn babies are oblivious to day and night and do not begin to develop circadian rhythms until about 2 months of age. However the breastfeeding mother's cycle of sleep/wake hormones transferred in her milk gradually influence her baby's circadian rhythm to develop.

Environmental cues of the morning and evening activities help establish baby's rhythm in sync with the family over time. Having baby's bassinet or pram located in the hub of the household during the day and exposed to family sounds and activities is beneficial to baby's sensory experience. Reducing stimulation during and after night feeds will assist baby to settle sooner after being fed. Close proximity to his parents will help baby settle until the next feed.

BABY'S DAY AND NIGHT PATTERNS

A COMMONLY RECOMMENDED PATTERN of caring for baby is "Feed, play, sleep". Although this pattern of feeding and sleep may suit some older babies (over 3 months of age) it is not biologically appropriate for young babies. A grizzly baby is often communicating a hunger for milk or sensation, or both. This is because young babies' neurological and digestive systems are immature and they often need another nappy change and the opportunity to feed again before "sleep pressure" takes over and baby naturally falls asleep.

It's quite Ok to wake your young baby to feed during the daytime if he does not self-waken after four hours or so have passed since his last feed. Avoiding long sleeps in the daytime will ensure baby has a consistent food intake through the day. Most babies will naturally have a longer sleep at some time during the 24 hours of each day, and if feeds and naps are frequent through the day he may be more likely to have the longer stretch of sleep during the night time hours. This often occurs in the early part of the evening, so be prepared to go to bed early yourself to maximise the benefits.

Night feeds are normal and necessary for baby's health and wellbeing. Giving baby a feed late in the evening (before midnight) can enhance the chance that baby may sleep for a few more hours after midnight. Sometimes called a "rollover feed" or "dream feed" the aim is to feed baby with minimal disturbance, however a nappy change should be done prior to the feed to waken baby enough to feed safely. Baby should never be fed by bottle when he is asleep, and bottle feeding a sleepy baby while laid in his bed is very dangerous as he may cough and aspirate milk into his lungs. All babies, whether bottle fed or breast fed, need to feed frequently and regularly around the clock to sustain the rapid physical and developmental growth that is constantly taking place.

Baby's sleep patterns change as they grow, and weary parents can be assured their baby will gradually sleep more at night as she matures. A study in Japan tracked babies' sleep patterns for the first 6 months of life. They found that in the early weeks of baby's life they were as likely to be awake at night as in the day. Around 7 weeks of age most babies were sleeping more at night than they were in the day. By twelve weeks most babies were having daytime naps and sleeping for a longer period of time during the night, but most were still waking for a feed at night. All babies are individuals and live in all sorts of family situations, however the patterns revealed by the Japanese study are fairly reflective of most babies in the early months.

Parents may crave order and predictability, hoping to "get into a routine" from birth. Knowing patterns appear naturally as baby develops physically and mentally will help them to adapt to their new lifestyle. This does not mean baby is dictating the terms of existence forever, it means the parents are meeting their baby's needs responsibly and sensitively as their new family becomes a cohesive functioning unit.

Following the highly structured and inflexible routines offered by "sleep trainers" is a one-size-fits-all concept which lock parents into rigid timeframes too. The self-proclaimed 'sleep experts' do not know or adjust for the baby's or the family's unique story. When something happens which confounds the 'routine' the parents are challenged to somehow get back on track, adding to their anxiety and a sense of failure if their baby does not "fit" into the prescribed routine.

A very comprehensive systematic review was published in the *Journal of Developmental & Behavioural Pediatrics* in 2013 which studied *Behavioural Sleep Interventions* (ie **sleep training**) in baby's first 6 months of life. They found that *"behavioural interventions in the first 6 months do not decrease infant crying, (or) prevent sleep and behavioural problems in later childhood, or protect against postnatal depression."* These authors concluded that *"parental empowerment is supported by education about sensible cue-based care, about healthy daytime biopsychosocial rhythms, and by addressing parental sleep anxiety, safe sleep, normal crying and unsettled infant behaviour."*

The Australian Infant Mental Health Association states: *"Infants are more likely to form secure attachments when their distress is responded to promptly, consistently and appropriately. Secure attachments in infancy are the foundation for good adult mental health."*

Health professionals now recognise there are potential hazards for baby's physical and mental development associated with rigid feeding routines and sleep training. Cue-based responsive parenting enhances baby's wellbeing and parents' confidence in caring for and understanding their baby's changing needs. For expert guidance about baby's sleep visit these excellent resources: **https://possumsonline.com/ https://www.pinkymckay.com**

BABY'S SLEEP ENVIRONMENT

BABY NEEDS A SAFE PLACE TO SLEEP and it is strongly recommended by SIDS experts that baby sleeps in the same room as his parents for the first 6 months of life. Most new babies sleep in a bassinet on a stand with wheels so you can move baby around the house as needed. Alternately baby could also sleep in a cot made up according to safe sleep recommendations (no bumper pads, pillows or quilts) with baby put at the bottom of the cot. The disadvantage of this option is that it is not easily moved if desired. Sleeping baby in a pram in the daytime and his cot in the parents' room at night is a good alternative.

Most parents are likely to take their baby into bed with them at some times for feeding or cuddles to settle, and maybe to sleep. Research indicates that mothers who co-sleep will breastfeed baby to an older age than mothers who do not co-sleep. If parents plan to have baby sleeping with them in their bed there are some important considerations to ensure this is done safely. Babies should never be slept in the same bed as a parent who smokes as the dangerous fumes exhaled by a smoker are passively breathed in by the baby. Smoking significantly increases the risk of cot death.

To prevent baby from becoming overheated or suffocating the bed should have a firm mattress, and not be positioned against any wall where baby could become entrapped. Baby should not be overdressed and baby should not be swaddled if sleeping beside an adult. Pillows and doonas should be moved well away from baby, and baby's own blanket tucked around him to avoid the parents bedding overheating baby or accidentally covering baby's face. Anyone else sharing the bed must know where baby is positioned, and pets should not be allowed to share the bed with a baby. Obese parents or anyone who is under the influence of alcohol or drugs should never sleep in bed with a baby. Baby sleep accidents occur most frequently when parents are co-sleeping on a sofa, couch or chair, so this is a very dangerous practice to avoid.

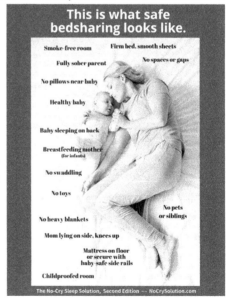

This is what safe bedsharing looks like.

Smoke-free room
Firm bed, smooth sheets
Fully sober parent
No spaces or gaps
No pillows near baby
Healthy baby
Baby sleeping on back
Breastfeeding mother (for infants)
No swaddling
No toys
No pets or siblings
No heavy blankets
Mom lying on side, knees up
Mattress on floor or secure with baby-safe side rails
Childproofed room

The No-Cry Sleep Solution, Second Edition — NoCrySolution.com

Source: *The No Cry Sleep Solution* (Second Edition, 2020) – **NoCrySolution.com**

A safe option for co-sleeping is one of the little baby beds designed for this purpose, such as The First Years - *Safe and Secure bed* or Sweet Dreams - *My Little Bed*. These are designed to give baby a safe sleep space in the parents' bed, away from their pillows and covers. Baby can be swaddled and tucked into his own little bed similar to a bassinet, but still be right beside his mother within easy reach for feeding and settling. Upright sides on the bed keep parents' bedding separate from baby, and a flap at the head of the little bed tucks firmly under the parents' mattress to keep it securely in place. The little bed can also be used inside a cot to assist the transition from a bassinet, and it folds up to be taken with you if going out with baby. These are readily available at baby shops and department stores. There are many bassinets which can be attached to the side of the parents' bed which also convert to a freestanding bassinet.

Once your baby's sleep zone is decided there are some simple strategies parents can employ to help baby to feel secure and relaxed in his bed. In the cooler months it can be very helpful to settle baby in a pre-warmed bed. This is simply a matter of putting a warm heat pack in his bed shortly before you lay him down so his sheets are warm and the transition from your arms is less noticeable. Always check the bed is not too hot and remove the heat pack before putting baby down. This can work especially well after night feeds.

Ensuring baby is fed and his nappy is dry before settling him will always be helpful. Baby's clothing should be soft and roomy so they do not restrict blood flow and his ability to stretch, and baby only needs one more layer of clothing on than you are wearing to be comfortably warm.

Most babies enjoy being swaddled which reminds them of the confined safe environment of the womb. Using a light cotton or muslin wrap to swaddle baby will provide the feeling of security without overheating baby, and additional wraps or blankets can be added if the room is very cool. Baby's hips legs should always be wrapped more loosely than his upper body. See the New Baby 101 **video "How to swaddle your baby"** for suggested wrapping techniques.

Another option are the various 'swaddle suits' which are like sleeping bags which close securely around baby's upper body keeping his arms inside. Some Mums find these easier and more effective than wrapping or swaddling baby. SIDS/RedNose have advised against using swaddle suits designed to position baby's arms raised upwards as they are regarded as risky if baby turns or rolls over, and concerns that restriction of arm movement could impede gross motor development and affect midline orientation. (Source: SIDS Education on-line forum 2021)

As babies grow and begin to move around more while asleep a sleeping bag may be another option to consider. Sleeping bags limit baby's ability to kick off his blankets and even if he does wriggle around he stays warm because the sleeping bag goes with him. Never use sleeping bags which have a hood attached as baby can quickly become overheated, which increases the risk of SIDS.

SETTLING STRATEGIES

SLEEP TRAINERS MAY ADVISE PARENTS to strictly adhere to certain bedtime rituals performed in a certain order at certain times of the day, however I believe it is a good idea to familiarise baby with a few different ways to prepare for sleep which can be helpful at any time of the day. Babies respond to their needs being met rather than a rigid series of actions to enable sleep to follow. Responding appropriately when baby tires is the most important message to take on board.

Any of the following sleep strategies can be utilised any time to enhance a young baby's relaxation and readiness for sleep. Firstly, ensure baby is comfortable with a dry nappy and comfortable clothes. Feed baby if he is hungry and if he falls straight to sleep - good for you! He will not be 'spoiled' by this action and don't worry if baby falls asleep without burping. Ensuring he feels secure by swaddling then holding baby and rocking gently in arms or in a sling until she becomes drowsy will help sleep to follow. You can put baby in his bed when drowsy or cuddle him until he is in a deeper sleep. There really are no rules so do what suits you and your baby.

If baby enjoys movement to relax a baby swing or pram can be used. Warming his bed if the environment is cool will make the transition away from the adult body easier. Patting baby gently and rhythmically when laid in his bed can provide comforting repetitious movement which can lull a drowsy baby off to sleep. Reassurance can also be provided by a familiar voice repeating a bedtime phrase or sung lullaby, some soft background music, or 'white noise' provided by an appliance like a fan. "Safe Sleep Space" have developed a CD for this purpose: **https://www.safesleepspace.com.au** Experiment with strategies which remove obstacles to sleep, and choose what suits the time, place and situation.

Giving baby his bath in the early evening can be a nice way for parents to share some time with baby, as long as it is a relaxing wind-down time. Giving baby a massage after a bath naturally increases baby's melatonin levels aiding her transition to drowsiness and sleep. Newborns may also benefit from having a massage as part of their **active alert** state *before* a bath, so they can enjoy the visual interaction with their parent. Following the massage with their bath can enhance deep relaxation and drowsiness enabling an easy transition to sleep.

However, in many households the early evening is the busiest time of the day, so baby's bath might be better planned for the mid-afternoon, particularly if baby has an unsettled time during the late afternoon which is typical of babies between 3 weeks and two months of age. If this is the case a handy way of drying an unsettled baby after bathing is to have two towels one on top of the other, and wrap baby in both towels and cuddle her. She will dry and relax while being cuddled and can even have a breast feed this way. Then baby can be laid down and all her folds and creases dried with the dry outer towel. Baby can then be dressed and complete the feed, and may now be comfortable and content ready for some quiet time and sleep.

Many older babies enjoy a dummy to suck as they go off to sleep. Keeping the dummy in baby's bed will help baby associate the dummy with sleep, rather than an awake-time 'plug' to keep him quiet.

EXPECT CHANGES

REMEMBER THAT BABY'S SLEEP patterns will change from time to time associated with growth spurts and developmental phases (sometimes called "wonder weeks") so don't despair if your settling strategies that worked for weeks suddenly don't work, and baby resists sleeping when she has slept easily in the past. Flexibility is the answer to these times of change and will save parents many wasted hours trying unsuccessfully to coax a baby to sleep when it is just not what she needs. More often than not these unsettled times are driven by hunger, and more feeding will be the answer to the situation because baby's nutritional requirements are in a state of change in response to growth. If baby does not need to feed, she simply won't. Next try a strategy involving movement – pram/stroller, car, swing, rocking in arms. In the end it is a case of *'try this, try that',* but always give the new strategy at least 15 minutes before moving to another settling strategy. It often takes that amount of time for baby to 'reset' and respond by calming down.

Take some deep breaths, close your eyes and relax yourself in order to recharge your own energy, and focus on your lovely little person. All parents experience these challenges at some time, it is part of the parenthood deal. If you are finding it very hard to cope with a wakeful baby talk about it with your Child Health Nurse or GP. Don't despair, help is nearby **https://possumsonline.com/ https://www.pinkymckay.com**.

Safety Tip – Amber necklaces for babies have become popular over recent years as some believe they reduce pain associated with teething. These necklaces are made from Baltic amber which is found in northern Europe. It's not a stone, it is fossilized tree sap that has been cultivated and polished. Baltic amber contains 3 to 8 percent of a substance called succinic acid which, when warmed by the skin, some believe relieves pain. There is no scientific evidence to support this, and amber necklaces have been identified as a choking risk following several tragedies. If used, **the necklace should be removed when baby is sleeping**, and the safest design has a magnetic clasp which releases if accidentally caught on something. There are fakes on the market too - real amber will float if placed in water.

Reference: *Journal of Developmental & Behavioural Pediatrics, "Behavioural Sleep Interventions in the First Six Months" Douglas PS, Hill PS, Vol 34, No7*, September 2013.

TOPIC 9
Fun Times

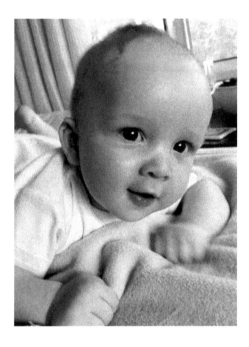

HUMAN BABIES HAVE immature physical and neurological functionality compared to other mammals whose newborns need to be able to stand and run beside or cling on to their mothers for safety from birth. Nevertheless, our human babies are responsive to lights and sounds, cold and warmth, hunger and pain which they experience as soon as they are apart from their quiet watery warm womb environment.

What can baby see? Newborn babies can see a distance of about 30cm – equivalent to the distance of a babe held in arms gazing at an adult's face. They have acute hearing and startle readily at loud noises. They are particularly attracted to studying faces (real or pictures) and closely observe facial expressions. Young babies can mimic some facial movements such as poking out their tongue when they see another person do the same. They also have a heightened sense of smell and recognise the scent of their mother and her colostrum and breastmilk, so it is advisable for Mothers to avoid wearing perfumes or strongly scented cosmetics in the early weeks of bonding with their new baby. In these early weeks of adjusting to their new world young babies' needs are very simple – food, warmth and comfort, and sleep.

Nevertheless, during their **quiet alert** state which usually occurs just before or closely following a feed they are most responsive to interaction opportunities to visually explore their world. Babies also "hunger" for sensory input – touch, pressure, movement, scents, sounds and warmth of skin and of course suckling associated with feeding, which are essential for healthy neuronal (brain) development. Breastfeeding AND bottle feeding can provide sensory nourishment via eye contact, soothing words and caresses, and responsiveness to baby's cues of hunger and satiety. Their most important source of sensory experience is you – their caregiver.

Using a baby carrier (preferably in an upright position) provides closeness for comfort as needed, but also physical movement and a change of view of their little world, which can be especially helpful when baby is unsettled. These times of exploration and experience are very important for baby's understanding of their surroundings and their security within it, assisting their adjustment to the rhythms of their home environment.

There is an enormous range of baby rockers, bouncers and swings available which can provide a handy source of entertainment and sensory experience for baby, while offering Mother an opportunity to briefly tend to her own needs. However, paediatric physiotherapists warn that <u>prolonged periods</u> "packaged" in a baby container of some kind should be avoided, especially using them for sleep. The "packaged baby phenomenon" where baby is rotated between travel capsule, rocker, swing and capsule with minimal time laid flat to play, rest or sleep has been shown to be detrimental to baby's physical development.

Forget "feed, play, sleep". We now know so much more about babies' neurological, nutritional and sensory needs. This out-dated mantra of parenting disregards the biological normality of babies "feeding to sleep".

The concept is still "out there" in older resources, and parents may continue to be advised to disregard their baby's needs when adopting this ritualistic feeding pattern. I once saw a mother of a 2 day old baby holding her grizzling, wiggling hungry baby in front of her face, jiggling her up and down, ignoring her feeding cues because she insisted it was her play time, not her feed time. True story! Young babies are naturally inclined to fall asleep after feeding, especially if breastfeeding. A more likely pattern to occur may be "feed, sleep, wake, nappy change/play, feed, sleep."

Baby's interactions - can take many forms and are not limited to your facial expressions and your voice, although these are most likely to become your primary "tools" for inviting baby's response. Touching and stroking baby's skin, particularly on the most sensitive zones of the hands, feet and mouth will stimulate baby and elicit a response. Cuddling baby gives him a message of closeness and containment, similar to when he was confined in the womb and is usually a relaxing and reassuring way of communicating with your baby. Baby massage is a delightful method of combining face to face communication with comforting physical sensory experience.

If baby is not enjoying the interactions he may arch his back or turn his face away from you, signalling to you he needs some space rather than closeness at that moment in time. Parents need to respect this "give me some space" cue. If baby turns away from a face he has been studying closely he is giving himself some 'time out' because he is becoming a bit overwhelmed. It is important to allow this very natural response and not turn baby around or follow him to renew the eye contact. He will return to the interaction when he feels ready.

The chemistry of face to face interaction is an automatic and instinctive response for the baby and for the adult involved. When we smile at a baby our pupils dilate – a sign that the sympathetic nervous system is pleasurably aroused. When baby sees the smiling face and dilated pupils his sympathetic nervous system is also automatically aroused. His pupils also dilate and his heart beats faster. The adult recognises baby's positive response and engages more with the baby. Two natural "feel good" chemicals called neuropeptide and dopamine are released from the brains of both the adult and the baby. These chemicals stimulate brain development and new tissue growth as well as creating a sense of wellbeing and pleasure, so adults and babies are more likely to respond positively to future interactions. I guess this is why strangers can't help looking into prams to talk to babies even if they don't know the parents!

Sounds babies like - Babies are very responsive to sounds and particularly voices. Speaking to baby in a calm soft voice with comforting words, or bright happy phrases during nappy changes, during and after feeds will feed baby's sensory need to engage positively with the world around him. A gentle voice singing softly when settling baby down towards sleep will have a calming effect. Babies enjoy music and songs, and lullabies have always been a mainstay of parents' comforting techniques over the years. Studies have revealed babies have 'music processing receptors' that are present in different areas of the brain, and activation of these receptors is beneficial for calming an aroused state in the infant's brain. Baby can and will tune-in to angry, loud voices and discord can be uncomfortable and frightening to baby, leading to unsettled behaviours.

Much discussion about overstimulation appears in parenting magazines and baby care books. The temperaments of babies vary, and some can cruise through a very stimulating situation without becoming irritable or overwhelmed, while others who are more sensitive to stimuli will clearly signal they 'want out' of an uncomfortably busy environment to which they have been exposed. Visits to shopping centres, groups of visitors all absorbed with the new baby at once, or being "played with" when baby has passed the quiet alert stage and is becoming drowsy or fussy can result in baby being temporarily uncomfortable and overwhelmed with their environment. Parents soon learn how to read their baby's cues and respond by "turning down" the stimulation dial to adjust baby's immediate environment - reconnecting with baby in a calm and reassuring way, and comforting baby with a nappy change or feed as needed.

TUMMY TIME

IT IS GOOD FOR BABY TO HAVE short periods of time on his tummy, a few times per day. For newborns this may only be a matter of seconds before they signal they are uncomfortable. Holding baby facing you and resting on your chest while seated is tummy time!

A convenient time to offer a little tummy time can be when baby's nappy is changed. Baby can be turned over onto his tummy and positioned so he can see your face for a little talk and view of the world from a different perspective. The benefit of tummy time is to build strength in the neck and upper body, assisting baby to raise his head, although young babies will do a lot of 'face planting' during these closely supervised times and an adult will move bub as soon as she's had enough of that position. Baby can then be turned over onto her back for a change of scenery. Tummy time can also be done on a bed with the adult sitting on the floor opposite baby's face, or on the floor with an adult laid nearby.

Staying with baby helps him feel safe and also ensures the time is not extended so long that he becomes upset or tired. Thirty to sixty seconds per session is plenty to begin with for a newborn. As baby grows and begins developing core stability and integrating muscle movement and strength in the upper back, shoulders and neck, the periods of tummy time can gradually be extended according to baby's ability to cope comfortably with that position. Having a few toys or safe objects in front of baby's view will encourage him to focus and reach towards them as he gets older. Tummy time provides opportunities to develop the skills and strength to move himself around in a circle, and roll over from front to back, and later from back to front when he is ready. Baby should not be placed on his tummy to sleep at any age.

All babies cry. It is normal, and it is their main means of communication. New parents often get very anxious about baby crying and can exacerbate the situation if they too over-react to baby's expression of discomfort or discourse. It is very common for babies to go through a rough patch of frequent crying between the ages of about 3 to 8 weeks, and this period is understood to be aligned with profound developmental changes. These times of frequent and sometimes prolonged crying may be described as "colic" or "unsettled periods". Whatever name you give this phase it is a tough time for everyone around, and provides an opportunity for rapid upskilling of parents as they develop their settling and comforting skills.

In the past some 'experts' recommended managing this period of excessive crying and fussing by limiting the baby's life to a darkened quiet room, where all feeds and care is carried out in isolation from stimuli. This was thought to enable baby's body chemistry to 'reset' and adjust to being able to cope with normal daily environmental stimuli again.   However, a recent study published in *The Journal of Developmental & Behavioural Pediatrics* revealed this practice limits the caregiver's ability to develop a healthy daytime bio-psychosocial rhythm, and diverse sensory stimulation not only optimises infant neurodevelopment but is associated with more settled infant behaviour when combined with cue-based care.   This is "medico-speak" for the sensible practise of keeping baby nearby during daily activities of life, inside and outside, and for parents to learn to make sense of baby's cues during his various sensory experiences.

Exploring the world - Babies are naturally interested in their surroundings, and explore their bodies and everything else within view and reach which is a vital part of growing and learning. As your baby discovers how things around her look, feel smell and sound she is developing her senses. Everything is new so there is no need to swamp baby with toys that do all sorts of tricks.

Other opportunities for visual stimulation are everywhere – watching the washing flap on the clothes line, the trees swaying in the wind or the jingle of windchimes on the verandah all provide interesting objects for baby to experience. A walk outside in the arms of a caregiver, even just around your back yard, can be the "magic switch" needed to distract an unsettled baby from his discomforts, with a calming effect on everyone.

Play time comes as baby grows, and making funny faces at him, smiling and laughing, singing little songs with hand actions all become part of the grown-up's repertoire of baby amusements.   Toys which rattle and baby can hold, even momentarily, can be introduced quite early.   Be prepared for baby's grasp to be good but his movements to be jerky, so prevent him from hitting himself unexpectedly with toys he doesn't realise are now an extension of his arm.   Baby's movements in the first 8 weeks are involuntary or reflexes, but as baby grows all these things are likely to go into baby's mouth so be careful what is offered to baby for play and discovery. Floor play mats with pictures and textured fabrics to explore on the base provide visual and tactile experiences, and an arch that can hold a few interesting little objects suspended overhead will provide all the extra entertainment a young baby needs during the early months of play time. A mirror with safe edges positioned for baby to see himself can be a source of fascination and exploration. Many babies enjoy holding or stroking soft or shiny fabrics between their fingers while drifting off to sleep.

Around two months of age baby really gets purposeful with her leg actions and he may enjoy kicking furiously in the bath or when having "no nappy time". It will be about three months before baby will become engrossed in her hands and feet and begin to reach towards your face or a toy, or grab at her own feet when they come into view. For a few weeks baby's favourite toy will be his/her feet!

Pets - If you have pets in the house you need to be very careful how you introduce them to your baby. No matter how well behaved your pet may be a new baby is a curious addition to their domain and it is possible they may become jealous of the newcomer who now gets a lot of the attention that was previously theirs. Giving your pet an item of clothing or fabric which has the scent of the new baby on it will help the pet to become familiar with the baby as part of the family and accept him more readily than if he has just been excluded from the scene completely.

Also try to keep your pet's routine the same after baby arrives, for example enlist someone to walk the dog regularly, so life goes on as normal for everyone. As baby grows he may grab and squeeze your pet when he is within reach and the pet's natural reaction could be really dangerous for baby. If in doubt, keep the pet OUT; interactions between baby and pet must be closely controlled and always supervised.

Milestones - Babies develop physically at their own pace and parents really can't speed up these natural milestones by intervening or helping. Your baby is a unique little individual and you will grow to love every gurgle, smile, squeak and "bottom-burp" he makes. I have already made the point that you are his most important and valuable source of entertainment, and he will become yours without a doubt. Another great resource for your ongoing parenting journey relating to your baby and his developmental milestones can be found on the Australian Parenting Website **www.raisingchildren.net.au**

The Fourth Trimester - The early months with your new baby is a precious time when parents are discovering a new dimension of their capacity for love. They are forming deep and lasting relationships and enriching their lives as a couple and a new family. This time passes very quickly, so my advice is to embrace and enjoy this blur of minimal sleep and maximum joy. I trust you have found New Baby 101 to be a helpful guide as you negotiate the steep learning curve of parenthood.

Special Thanks to Sally Hicks
www.marvilloso.com.au
for providing her beautiful images
for the pages of New Baby 101,
and Megan Willis Photography
whose client_____

permitted use of their photo for the cover.

DEDICATION
– To Mothering

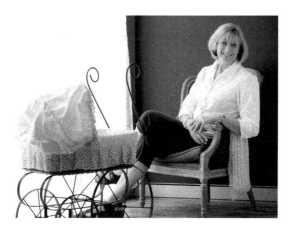

THIS BOOK IS DEDICATED to my eldest sister, Val. The week that my first baby was due to be born our dear mother died after a year-long battle with cancer. Mum's illness was very much our family's focus during my pregnancy, and Val had borne the lion's share of caring for Mum during that difficult and sad year.

When my new son Joseph was born I was just 20 years old. I had been married for two years, and my husband's family welcomed their first grandchild with love and enthusiasm. Val, a single mum of three teenagers, slipped effortlessly and naturally into the role that my own Mother would have loved to fulfil.

Val guided me practically and gently through the steep learning curve of new motherhood. Val always knew what to do, how to do it, and turned up when I needed her most throughout my mothering journey - which culminated in three babies in four years (which I do not recommend, but survived!)

So, thanks to my "Big Sis" - one of the great blessings of my lifetime. This book is dedicated to your skilful mothering and endless love. Lois

Footnote: Val passed away in May 2013. Rest in Peace.

INDEX

.

CPSIA information can be obtained
at www.ICGtesting.com
Printed in the USA
LVHW010105020422
714993LV00009B/514

9 780645 393811